MORE ~~DS

Cancer and the Dirty Electricity Plague

THE MISSING LINK ...

DONNA FISHER

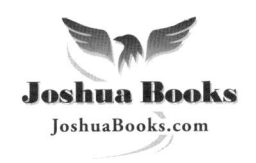

Joshua Books
JoshuaBooks.com

Joshua Books
PO Box 1668
Buddina 4575
Queensland Australia

© Copyright Donna Fisher

First Printed 2009

The right of Donna Fisher to be identified as the author of this work has been asserted by her in accordance with the Copyright, Designs and Patents act.

All rights reserved. No part of this publication may be reproduced, stored in or introduced into a retrieval system, or transmitted, in any form, or by any means (electronic, mechanical, photocopying, recording or otherwise) without the prior written permission of the publisher. Any person who does any unauthorised act in relation to this publication may be liable to criminal prosecution and civil claims for damages.

This book is an educational document outlining an important, emerging public health issue. It is not to be construed as medical advice. For individual health issues please see your physician or other licensed health practitioner.

Whilst every care has been taken to provide current reliable information based on scientific data, the publisher accepts no liability for any errors or omissions that may be present in this book, and no liability is accepted arising directly or indirectly as a result of reading or other use of this book.

ISBN 978 0 9806061 1 9

Category: Health: Educational: Author: Title

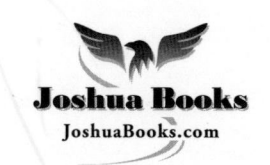

Joshua Books
JoshuaBooks.com

This book is dedicated to the many scientists who have worked so diligently on their research in the quest to help humanity. History has shown that the bravest, whether they are scientists or engineers in the areas that challenge current beliefs, are often ostracised and their credibility shattered.

It is indeed a humbling experience to be able to spread this information. I have been privileged in that the people dedicated to the research in this area have given me their time and answered my persistent questions, answers to which throw up yet more questions. I hope I have done justice to their work.

Donna

ACKNOWLEDGEMENTS

I extend my heartfelt thanks to James Alward. Without your support and encouragement to keep working on the challenging task of writing *Silent Fields: The Growing Cancer Cluster Story: When Electricity Kills*, which is helping so many, that first book would never have been published. Thank you for offering the services of Geoff Robin, who also played a pivotal role in the completion of *Silent Fields*, and thank you for offering me a sanctuary in which to write *More Silent Fields*.

I also thank Phillip Enkelmann for helping me with this book. You understood, many years ago, and I know you share my passion for spreading the message globally that electromagnetic radiation is killing some and making others very sick.

ABOUT THE AUTHOR

Donna Fisher loves a challenge and her very first one came early. At the tender age of four, like millions of children worldwide she started school. Having stuttered on every letter since she first spoke, reading in class was torture. Stuttering can become so serious that it makes a vocational failure of even a talented person, but not in Donna's case. She overcame her disordered speech after years of effort and today her stutter is mild and infrequent. She asserts, with great determination, that she will gain complete fluency.

After leaving school Donna involved herself in many worthy causes and successful commercial enterprises, but it wasn't enough to satisfy her drive, energy and restlessness. After studying transpersonal psychology, she attended an intensive workshop on leadership and went on to complete a thesis with special emphasis on the positive role of women in co-creating a better world.

In 1999, the first letter from the electric utility company arrived, alerting her to the issue of the invisible fields from electricity being a concern. Donna's increasing comprehension of owning her own mind combined easily with her patient nature, leading her to study the attributes of the 'Warrior Path' and the ways in which change can come through peaceful means. She volunteered shortly after that to work for eighteen months for a non-profit association dealing with child abuse.

When Donna took on the case against the power company she had long learned that the way forward for all of personkind is through sharing reality in a co-creative way, and the way forward for her personally was by intervening with positive action on issues that were particularly important to her. She believes that by claiming and owning one's mind, humanity can live intelligently through the heart; while a little knowledge can be dangerous, too much knowledge takes away the heart sense.

Born in Australia, Donna has an international following and is also involved in promoting her books and, with the help of a dedicated team, chairs Donna Fisher Silent Fields Inc, through which she offers practical solutions for 'cleaning' electricity. While there is a touch of the crusader in Donna, this energetic person does not invade your privacy but encourages you, albeit with great passion, to protect yourself and your family against the dirty electricity plague.

CONTENTS

1	Electricity and Disease	11
2	Cancer and Dirty Electricity	27
3	The Missing Link	33
4	Diabetes	43
5	Dirty Electricity and Breast Cancer	47
6	The Wireless Revolution	57
7	The Venice Resolution	67
8	Autism	71
9	Genes versus Environment	81
10	Cancer Treatment Using Radiowaves	91
11	What You Can Do	95
12	Cleaning Up Electricity	99
	Afterword	109
	Appendix A: Electromagnetic Frequencies	115
	Appendix B: Legal Advice to the Power Industry	117
	Appendix C: For the Technically Minded	119
	Appendix D: How Clean is Our Lighting?	123
	Appendix E: Signees to the Venice Resolution	129
	Resources	133
	Glossary	135
	Bibliography	139
	Notes	143

CHAPTER 1

Electricity and Disease

In my campaign to clean up electricity, the struggles and challenges that I face on a daily basis continue. The premise that the silent and invisible electromagnetic fields (EMFs) from electricity could kill and make others very sick has been met with shock by some, but many people unable to trace the cause of their illnesses finally find relief when exposure to these fields created from electricity is lessened.

CASE HISTORY #1

A sixty-six year old woman in generally good health complained of a nine-year history of debilitating daily headaches and intermittent dizziness. Neurological assessment was unremarkable and a computer tomography scan, magnetic resonance imaging and electroencephalogram were reported normal.

At a chronic-pain clinic, the patient received narcotic analgesics and a diagnosis of 'primary pain disorder'. Detailed aetiological history was unremarkable, other than the patient used an electric toothbrush six times a day for meticulous care of failing dentition. Gaussmeter assessment revealed inordinately high levels of EMFs (>200 mG units) emanating from the toothbrush. Within six weeks of discontinuing the use of her toothbrush, the headaches subsided and, with assistance, she was quickly able to overcome her dependence on prescription analgesics.

CASE HISTORY #2

A thirty-three year old woman wishing to have a large family complained of six consecutive pregnancy losses. After two uncomplicated pregnancies with vaginal deliveries, the patient changed residences and subsequently experienced three first-trimester miscarriages.

After assessments by a family physician, a gynaecologist, an infertility specialist and a specialty reproductive care unit, the patient subsequently sustained three second-trimester losses despite interventions, including clomiphene, human chorionic gonadotrophin injections, progesterone supplementation and counselling. According to her history, the only potential determinant that appeared to have changed from when she experienced the two completed gestations was her employment as a seamstress for six hours a day in the basement of her new residence, an environment with low ceilings and fluorescent lights.

Using a gaussmeter, the woman recorded high EMF levels (≥ 104 mG units) in the vicinity of her head when fluorescent lighting in her workplace was turned on, and high EMF levels (~180 mG units) adjacent to her sewing machine. Following advice to decrease EMR exposure by avoiding fluorescent lights and minimising the use of her sewing machine, the woman promptly conceived and carried the pregnancy to full term.

CASE HISTORY #3

A seventeen year old boy experiencing a three-year history of intrusive thoughts relating to religious themes believed he had committed unpardonable sins and was convinced the devil was imminently sending him to hell. As well as increasing depressive symptoms, the adolescent displayed escalating aggression towards his parents. The nominally religious parents took their son for religious counselling, to no avail. Psychiatric diagnosis included a thought disorder. Psychotropic medication failed to control the symptoms but caused numerous side effects.

Human exposure assessment uncovered extremely high gauss measurements ($\geq$ 200 mG units) at the head of the teen's bed, as electrical entry to the house was immediately adjacent to the bedroom, right beside his bed. He moved to another bedroom and all other sources of EMF exposure were minimised.

Within twelve weeks the intrusive thoughts had abated considerably, the mood symptomatology had declined, medication was stopped, and the parents indicated that their son was now a friendly, motivated boy. One episode of symptom aggravation subsequently occurred immediately following four hours of online work in a high school computer laboratory; those symptoms subsided within seventy-two hours of deliberate EMF avoidance. All adverse symptoms completely cleared within six months and wellness was maintained over the next two years and at the time of writing.[1]

I cannot emphasise enough that there is no safe level of exposure: 0 mG units is desirable, and levels of 2–4 mG units have been determined to be risky.[2]

CANCER CLUSTERS

After the release of my first book *Silent Fields: The Growing Cancer Cluster Story: When Electricity Kills*, the high incidence of breast cancer continued to haunt me as I walked the often difficult path in my stance that electromagnetic radiation, and our electrical environment in general, is a significant contributor to the dramatic rise in breast cancer, and is the reason for the breast cancer statistics being so high.

The incomplete investigation in Brisbane, Australia of the electrical environment at the Toowong ABC TV studios' breast cancer cluster prompted me to put pen to paper in *Silent Fields* to explain why seventeen women in one small area of a workplace developed breast cancer. This second book is the result of my dismay that the explanation of 'random chance' in regard to the increasing cancer clusters is still being used! Until the real culprit of cancer clusters is confronted, tragically the breast-cancer clusters will continue to occur.

For example, in late November 2008 Professor David Roder, head of research and information science at Cancer Council SA (South Australia), released a report into the investigation of the breast cancer cluster in Australia's Adelaide Women's and Children's Hospital.

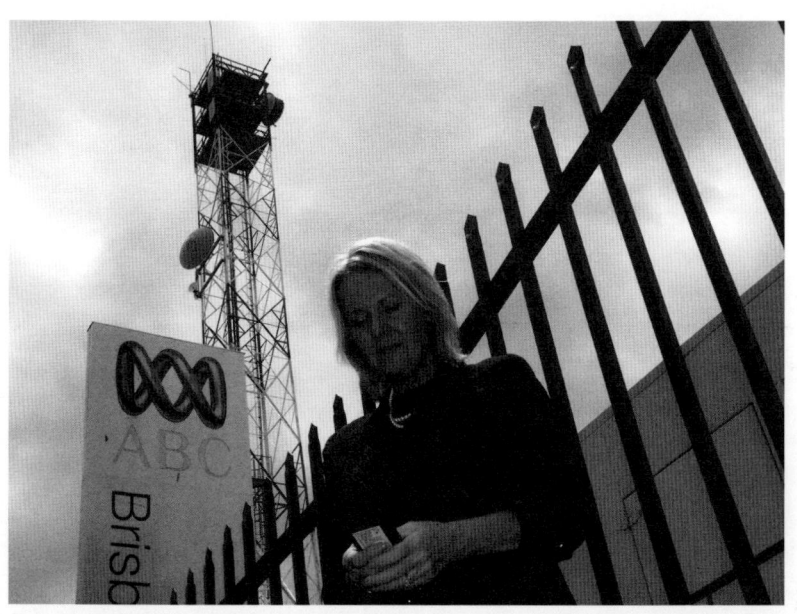

ABC TV STUDIOS: Measuring for dirty electricity can be a simple process

The maternity and neonatal care ward was the area of concern. Even though humidicribs can have very high levels of EMFs - a continuing area of cancer research - those caring for the infants can also be exposed to high EMFs.

Professor Roder found nine more cases than might normally occur in a workforce of a similar size, but he concluded that the higher than usual number was a random occurrence and there was no apparent causal environmental agent that could be linked to the elevated number of cases. It is just not good enough when so many people's lives are at stake. In 2008 the United States alone had 108 breast cancer clusters and Australia's figure is rising.

Explanations of 'random' and 'coincidence' occur far too frequently in an age where integrity must be a willing partner with science in addressing the growing cancer cluster story. It is not only fields from power lines and substations that are a concern: fields from the wiring in our homes, workplaces, schools and hospitals are of just as much concern.

LESSENING EXPOSURE TO EMFs

Consider a vulnerable child with or recovering from leukaemia—in fact, any person with cancer—in hospital being exposed to high measurements of these silent EMFs from medical equipment and wiring while they are awake, and particularly while healing as they sleep.

Consider a child at school, or a person spending long hours in their workplace, where the fluorescent lighting and wiring from the floor below are emitting high measurements of these silent EMFs beneath them. Consider people sleeping with the meter box on the other side of their bedroom wall or those who sleep with electrical equipment close to their heads. Promotional signs directly outside one's apartment or bedroom window can also yield high measurements of these EMFs.

Lessening our exposure to EMFs must become a way of life,

as exposure to these silent fields, combined with other toxic agents, has the ability to produce a deadly cocktail.

Following a study in 2006, scientists who had been concerned for decades called for a lowering of the exposure limits to these EMFs. An analysis of sixty-five studies reported that, compared to exposure to the toxic agent alone, the combined effect of toxic agents and these silent fields *enhanced* the damage.

For example, consider a hairdresser who is exposed to chemicals—some of which may be toxic agents—and who uses a hairdryer for a large part of the day. Although the client is sitting down, the hairdresser is standing and holding, at breast level, a hairdryer that emits very high measurements of these fields. If a measurement of 1.8 mG units has been indicated with childhood leukaemia, can you imagine what the average hairdryer, which emits 70 mG units, can do?

As another example of the danger of the combined effects of EMFs and possibly toxic agents, consider a pregnant female who stands in front of a photocopier or photo-developing machine for many hours a day, where exposure to high measurements of these fields is also a concern. And consider also the effect of the exposure to these fields combined with the possibly toxic chemicals emitted from the machine.

THE SMOKING LINK

Consider people who smoke. The chemical carcinogens in cigarette smoke cause 'DNA breaks' that damage our precious and life-giving DNA. Damaged DNA increases the risk of cancer. Similarly, exposure to EMFs has also been shown to cause DNA breaks.[3] So if you are a smoker, being exposed to both is a double hit! Cigarette-smoking and EMFs can both damage DNA on their own. EMFs can also enhance the toxic exposure from the cigarettes.

In January 2009 scientists at Cancer Institute NSW found that leukaemia, and brain, kidney and eye cancers are common in children whose mothers smoked during pregnancy, drawing for the first time a direct link with cancer. (The institute linked the records of all births in New South Wales between 1994 and 2005 with causes of cancer in children during the same period). Even though smoking during pregnancy has long been advised against, scientists have never before drawn a direct link with cancer. It is my hope that it does not take decades before the wisdom of avoiding direct exposure to EMFs while pregnant is common knowledge. Also, it would be wise for women to stop using a mobile phone when pregnant.

CAUSE AND EFFECT

When a report by the California Department of Health Services was released in 2002, legal counsel for the electrical industry worldwide conceded that the attitude of the power industry had to change. The belief of legal representatives for the power industry was that it would be 'legally inadvisable' to make a global statement that there is *no* cause-and-effect relationship between these fields and disease.[4]

The Russians have been protecting their citizens from these EMFs since the 1950s, and the Swedish government instigated measures in the 1990s. Denmark, Italy, Switzerland, Israel, the Netherlands and Slovenia are also in the process of implementing measures.

In June 2007 the World Health Organization concluded that reducing exposure to these silent EMFs—scientifically termed 'extremely low frequency electromagnetic fields' (ELF EMF)—from power exposure is reasonable and warranted, provided that the health, social and economic benefits of electric power are not compromised. This addresses the fields (magnetic) from 50/60 Hz wiring, which was the main focus of *Silent Fields*.

Sadly, this information will take many decades to filter around the world.

ANOTHER SIDE TO ELECTRICITY

With that determined, we now have another facet of electricity that is proving to be more perilous and more prevalent in our lives. Dirty electricity, another by-product of the generation of electricity, is an invisible and unwelcome character that relies on an already overloaded power system. (For more in-depth information on dirty electricity, see appendix C.)

The pioneer who cautioned on these fields, Dr Robert O Becker (twice nominated for a Nobel Prize in regard to the healing aspects of the fields) believed the increasing proliferation of electromagnetic fields to be a greater threat than global warming. Electromagnetic fields from electricity so concerned him that in 1990 he stated:

> ... it is quite possible that chronic exposure to these fields is a competent cause for the origin of cancers. This is compatible with the latest data indicating significant increases in the incidence of specific types of cancers since 1975. According to Dr Samuel Epstein of the University of Chicago Medical Center:
>
> - lymphoma, myeloma, and melanoma have increased by 100 percent,
> - breast cancer by 31 percent,
> - cancer of the kidney by 142 percent,
> - and colon cancer by 63 percent.[5]

The significance of such a dramatic rise in cancer since 1975 made me wonder what had happened to create this situation. One very important event, which had significant influence in our world, occurred back in the early 1970s.

During the oil embargo of 1973, manufacturers of equipment were forced to design products that would save energy. One method was to have the equipment draw current in an intermittent way instead of in a continuous flow. Unfortunately this created overloading of our wiring, resulting in the 'burning buildings' of the late 1970s and 1980s. The excess current on wiring that was not designed to handle this load caused fires. Because of this change in the mode of flow, i.e. going from a continuous to an intermittent electrical flow, something significant occurred. The change allowed for the creation of 'dirty electricity', an intermittent flow of electrical current that spikes into a dangerous higher frequency. These spikes, or surges, are technically termed 'high-frequency voltage transients' (I refer to them as transients and transient EMF).

Further to this revelation, I was fortunate enough to correspond with many of the leading specialists who were researching dirty electricity, which was an even more insidious menace than I had imagined. My continued research has now given me a greater understanding of why the incidence of breast cancer has increased so dramatically since the arrival of computers.

On 24 February 2009, the night before I was to submit this manuscript to my publisher, I came across an article just posted at *Microwave News*[6] regarding eight women who worked in the literature building at the University of California, San Diego (UCSD) campus. All eight women had developed breast cancer between 2000 and 2006. Cedric Garland, an epidemiologist at UCSD, reported that the number of breast cancer cases alone was significantly more than would have been expected by chance. In his report, he noted that the risk of invasive breast cancer for employees in the literature building appeared to be four to five times higher than that of the general Californian population. In his June 2008 report to Marye Anne Fox, UCSD chancellor and a professor of chemistry, Garland focused on the possible role played by EMFs, especially 'transients' - dirty electricity - from the motors of the building's elevators.

Finally, this is an issue whose time has come. As Shakespeare said, 'Truth is the daughter of time.' So, as simply as I can, I will continue to encourage awareness and work towards a world that is free of disease, where ethical behaviour towards cancer-cluster investigations is a priority, and prevention of disease is paramount.

In December 2008 the World Cancer Report, issued by the World Health Organization, noted that by 2010 cancer is expected to surpass heart disease as the world's leading cause of death, killing more people than the combined death toll from AIDS, malaria and tuberculosis.

Dirty electricity—another environmental assault that has woven itself into our societal structure—is a large part of the cancer, and growing cancer-cluster, story.

> **'... chronic exposure to these fields is a competent cause for the origin of cancers.'**
>
> —Dr Robert O Becker 1990, twice nominated for the Nobel Prize

HELEN'S STORY

Excessive Levels of Electromagnetic Radiation

Would you have any idea what your home's ambient background level of electromagnetic radiation (EMR) is? Would it mean anything to you if I said that during waking hours it should not be above 2 mG units? Probably not, but let me put this into perspective for you.

If this background level is raised to just 4 mG units, illness patterns begin to show up. Risk levels of childhood leukaemia go up at 4 mG. Between 6–12 mG units affects melatonin (hormone) levels sufficiently to stop breast cancer cells from repairing.

But first let me give a bit of background about myself. Newly married in 2002, my husband and I moved into an old Victorian home in Flemington. We lead a healthy lifestyle, we're vegetarian, don't drink or smoke, and my background includes studies in very alternative health fields, so it was puzzling to me when I began experiencing strange symptoms.

At first I couldn't understand the constant fatigue I was experiencing, but I put it down to wedding preparations and coming off shift work after ten years. I would try and have a nap on a Saturday afternoon, but would not fall into a deep sleep, rather a half-awake, half-asleep, dream-type state. In 2004 I began studying building biology, although not to solve my problems because I had not yet twigged to the cause, which was ironic. After learning a little about EMR, a subject that I did not begin until late 2005, I kept the information in the back of my mind.

Little things happened along the way to point me in the right direction. For instance, I was experiencing electrostatic shocks fairly often, and when I stayed in a country town motel late in 2004 my whole body felt like it was being zapped when I lay down on the bed with the electric blanket turned on.

At some stage I realised that at my work I had two computers pointing at my back from less than a metre away, protected only by a thin partition. Only metres away a room was buzzing with a bank of about sixty portable radios on charge. By this time I was having funny, fuzzy headaches, and I had never been one to get headaches. My constant fatigue led to erratic behaviour and mood swings, much to the dismay of my embattled husband, who wondered where his calm, collected wife had gone.

During this time we were also keen to conceive. Medical tests revealed that this was a sure probability, but it just wasn't happening. We sought help through several natural fertility methods and bingo! But our joy was to be short lived when I miscarried at ten weeks early in 2005. This was another legacy of high EMR levels, so I was to learn later.

In mid 2005 I began the electrobiology component of my course. My health by this time was getting progressively worse. I was experiencing severe joint pain, tinnitus, heart palpitations and more. My mental coherence capabilities were spiralling down and I am sure I was difficult to be around. However, the blessing of this component was the realisation of what was bringing on all these strange symptoms and weird behaviour.

I had just purchased my first piece of measuring equipment: a meter which could measure the EMR output of household electrical items and power fields. I tested it around the college and got a feel for its capabilities before trying it out at home.

When I did turn it on at home, my eyebrows raised and I thought, This can't be right, something's wrong here. I charged around the house with it, but the level of 12 mG units on a Saturday afternoon would not drop. In the next few weeks all the pieces began to fit together: the fatigue, the mental instability, the joint pain, and on it went.

I had become so electrically sensitive (ES) that driving under the E-tag gantry on the Citylink (Melbourne, Australia) caused stabbing pains in my heart, which would continue palpitating for up to five hours afterwards. The E-tag gantry device is run with microwave energy, similar to a mobile phone.

After three years of searching, I had finally found the culprit: two power poles emitting unusually high fields into my home. These were 50-Hz magnetic fields, as opposed to the many other EMR types.

Unfortunately there is no easy way of blocking magnetic fields, but after investing a lot of money and effort into renovating we were reluctant to leave. I then began trialling and testing many devices and ways of alleviating the majority of my symptoms by using a mix of devices, techniques and dietary supplements. This remains an ongoing process.

In my research, I came to understand that along with EMR fields of most types there is a component that is often termed 'dirty electricity'. When I measured my home's level of dirty electricity, I could trace the higher levels around appliances and electronic devices. I use them in a limited manner only, but overall, and because of the power lines' high emission into my home, the house had a toxic level of dirty electricity.

To counteract these emissions I used STETZERiZER filters that are specifically designed to lessen the toxic load of dirty electricity riding into the home through the power lines, wiring and electronic devices.

My first reaction was to notice how quiet my body felt from within. Having high magnetic fields constantly running through my body had made me feel like everything was very tense inside my muscles and I would often awaken in the night feeling my body vibrating with the electricity. Now, due to the absence of the tenseness, which began to feel normal after a while, I felt calmness come over me. I slept better and the joint pain that had been becoming disturbing quietened down too. I was later to learn that EMR runs through the bone marrow, creating inflammation and the breaking of calcium ion bonds.

My mental coherence improved again too. EMR and dirty electricity tends to have a scrambling effect on the mind and brain, which can be very debilitating. It is hard to get others to understand what is happening to you within when you appear normal outwardly, even though you are having such difficulty trying to piece a sentence together that the mind will not bring them forth, even when you know the words. And you cannot say them correctly either.

Interestingly, my dog Brigette, a 40-kg Briard, was also suffering from the magnetic fields and dirty electricity. Each remedy that I tried on me, I also tried on her. When I installed the filters, Brigette was eight years old and could hardly manage a walk around the block due to severe pain in her legs. To set the picture, she is a well-cared-for pet, eating mainly a diet of fresh butcher-shop meat and organic raw vegies. Her response was quite rapid and soon she was again walking several kilometres a day with me.

I was surprised but realised that this little-known phenomenon of dirty electricity certainly has an effect on human and animal bodies that is not acknowledged by many medical experts, scientists and, least of all, our electrical suppliers.

I have since tested many homes for levels of dirty electricity and have not yet found any to be sustained at optimal levels for health.

Now, in 2009, my health has returned to a level where I can function pretty normally mentally and physically, due to the implementation of the STETZERiZER filters and a raw-food diet.

This is what it takes to sustain my health under these conditions, even though it should not be so.

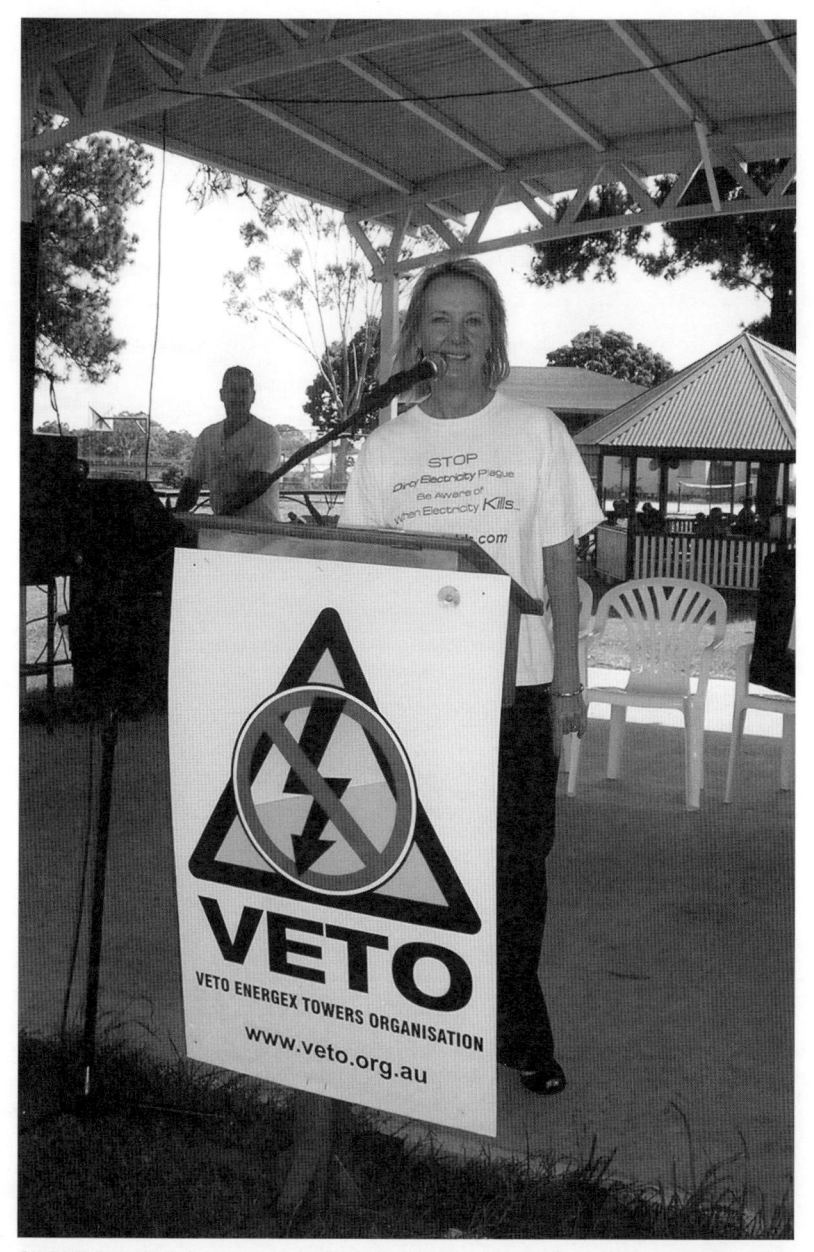

SILENT RALLY: It is not only the people fighting power lines that need to make a stand for their health—this issue affects everyone and we must all stand together.

CHAPTER 2

Cancer and Dirty Electricity

When two highly qualified leaders in their fields came out of retirement due to their concern for the people, new information worthy of creating a paradigm shift emerged. Even though the school district administration had refused a number of requests for these men to assist in the evaluation of a larger number of cancers reported by the teachers at La Quinta Middle School in California, a teacher invited these experts to visit the school after hours to take measurements of the electrical environment, which they did at their own expense.

When these researchers reported their findings to the superintendent of schools, the highly esteemed doctor was threatened with prosecution for 'unlawful ... trespass' and the teacher received a letter of reprimand. These brave men had honourable intentions and impressive credentials. Winner of the prestigious Ramazzini Award and the first to link workers exposed to EMFs with higher rates of leukaemia in 1982 Sam Milham MD MPH, while working with the Washington State Department of Health, conducted a study (2001) with E M Ossiander on the history of electrification of the UK and USA. They concluded that the childhood leukaemia peak of (cALL) was attributable to residential electrification: 75% of all childhood acute lymphoblastic leukaemia and 60% of all childhood leukaemia could be preventable. (It was reported as early as 1960 (Court-Brown and Doll) that a new leukaemia agent was introduced into the UK and USA in the 1920s and 1930s). L Lloyd Morgan BS an electronics engineer and a devoted pioneer in brain tumour research in regard to EMFs had been Director of the Central Brain Tumour Registry of the United States.

The teachers then filed a California OSHA complaint, which ultimately led to the California Department of Health Services becoming involved. The department measured the magnetic field (mG units) and dirty electricity (GS units) levels at the school, providing the exposure data for the La Quinta study. The courageous actions of these people and the interpretation of the data resulted in further validation of the missing link.

There had been only one study, in 1994, of dirty electricity in the Western world. Researchers at McGill University in Montreal, Canada published results showing that electric utility workers exposed to dirty electricity showed an increased incidence of lung cancer.[7] Further data was not able to be collected: the missing link, dirty electricity, was not welcome due to the enormous implications it had for society, and the power companies, and the implications regarding cancer and increasing disease.

LA QUINTA MIDDLE SCHOOL
LANDMARK CANCER CLUSTER STUDY

The second study of dirty electricity, now released to the world, is the 2008 landmark study of the cancer cluster at La Quinta Middle School. In the years 1988–2005, 137 teachers were employed at the school. On investigating the eighteen cancers in these teachers it was found there was a 1:10,000 possibility that this was due to chance. There were nearly three times more cancer cases than expected. The eighteen cancers in the sixteen affected teachers were:

- Four malignant melanomas
- Two female breast cancers
- Two cancers of the thyroid
- Two uterine cancers
- One Burkitt's lymphoma (a type of non-Hodgkins lymphoma)
- One polycythemia vera
- One multiple myeloma
- One leiomyosarcoma
- One cancer of the colon
- One cancer of the pancreas
- One cancer of the larynx

The critical finding was that the authors reported that the cancer incidence in the teachers at this school was unusually high and was strongly associated with dirty electricity that the authors state may be a universal carcinogen similar to ionising radiation[8], an established cause of cancer. Studies into ionising radiation, have shown an increased incidence in a number of different cancers. The study at La Quinta Middle School also showed an increase in the number of different cancers.

In the La Quinta Middle School study, all cancers had risk ratios that were statistically significant.

***What is most important is that the cancer risks at La Quinta Middle School are comparable to the cigarette smoking/lung cancer risks. There is no unexposed population.*[9]**

The authors noted that the relatively short latency time of melanoma and thyroid cancers suggests that these cancers may be more sensitive to the effects of high-frequency transients—dirty electricity/transient EMF—than the other cancers seen in this population.

How could dirty electricity create conditions to allow cancer to develop? Milham and Morgan postulated that the dirty electricity in the classroom wiring, which exerted its effect by capacitive coupling, induced electrical currents in the teachers' bodies. To explain this further, in addition to being part of an electrical circuit because of the electrical earth currents, each person is part of the transfer of energy within an electrical network to the wires running around them through the walls, floor, and ceiling of the building where they work or live.

It must be comprehended that a dirty electrical environment can create not only clusters of the same type of cancer but also a spread of different cancers in these clusters that have been silently occurring for decades. Cancer groupings are not just statistical anomalies of unrelated coincidences in a world full of cancer and a world in which a diagnosis of cancer is not seen as unusual. Dirty electricity is now seen as a major contributor to disease processes, individual cases of cancer and clusters of cancer.

Both leukaemia and brain tumours feature prominently in the growing cancer story in regard to electricity. The study also focused attention on Elgin-Millville High School in Minnesota, where a teacher who had taught in a room that had been tested for dirty electricity died of brain tumours. Another teacher in an adjoining room died of leukaemia. Both types of cancer feature prominently in the dirty electricity story.

To read the PDF of the complete study of the cancer cluster at La Quinta Middle School go to http://silentfields.com and click on Reports/Studies.

As Milham and Morgan reported that magnetic fields (mG units) showed no association with cancer incidence in this study by delving deeper into how dirty electricity is created and how it can play a role in cancer and disease states the culprits can be found in our everyday use of electrical equipment and appliances.

AN AUSTRALIAN SCHOOL

In late February 2009 an investigation began into the electromagnetic environment at Hazelwood School, Moonah, Tasmania. The school is close to transmission lines supplying power to a zinc smelter and has an electrical substation in the basement. There was excessive corrosion in the water pipes, which suggested electrical ground currents in the water system. Most significantly, the swimming pool had to be closed and drained because people were getting electrical shocks when entering the water.

The Department of Health and Community Services conducted a survey wherein detailed EMR measurements were carried out using new equipment to give a better idea of exposures in multiple locations in classrooms and offices over a period of time. EMR levels were reported as low. The Public and Environmental Health Service also looked for causal factors and environmental hazards.

Tasmanian EMR consultant Don Maisch of EMFACTS Consultancy offered his services free of charge. He has been watching this investigation closely and comments that the survey was conducted only *after* extensive electrical work was carried out at the school to rectify a major ground-current leakage problem that would have resulted in excessive magnetic fields in the building. According to a staff member—as reported by Don Maisch—about two weeks prior to this survey the Department of Education had extensive electrical work carried out at the school, including replacement of circuit boards. Maisch comments that it is interesting that the mitigation work was carried out just at the time the department was concerned that a former staff member was considering taking legal action.

Cancers among staff included breast (eight cases), colon, lung, skin, cervical and haemopoietic cancers (including lymphomas). These are cancers that feature quite prominently in environments with dirty electricity.

Maisch reports that students were not studied, in part because as a group they have a range of serious conditions. Some of their genetic conditions are already associated with a high risk of cancers, including leukaemia early in life. If EMR exposure is capable of exacerbating their predisposition, surely more could be done on a preventative level to ensure they are in a clean electrical/ electromagnetic environment.

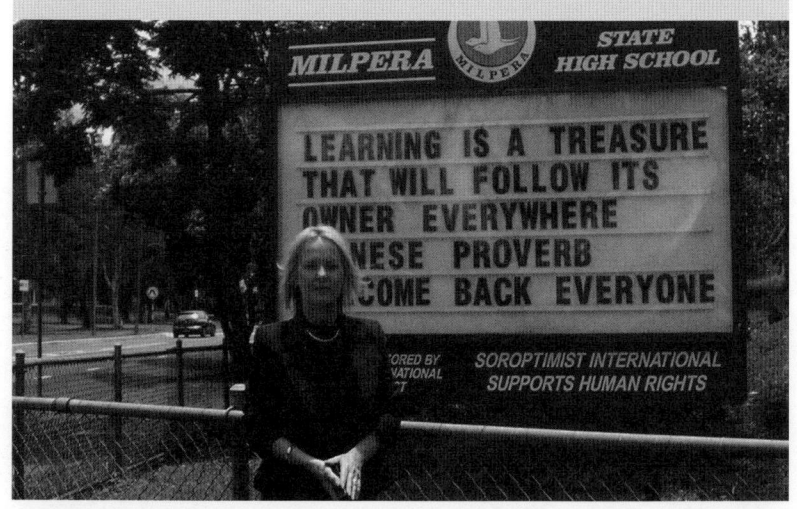

SEEKING TO HELP: The author offers information at Milpera School, Brisbane, Australia, where there is a suspected cancer cluster.

CHAPTER 3

The Missing Link

Power-quality expert Dave Stetzer, one of the leading experts in the field of dirty electricity in the United States, pooled information with leading specialists from Russia, Ukraine and Kazakhstan and together they conducted further research. They reported that there is a frequency range even more dangerous to humans than normal power frequency (50/60 Hz) and currently seen as more dangerous even than the much higher frequencies of our wireless and mobile telecommunications (800 MHz–2.5 GHz). The most studied area is 1 kHz–100 kHz. Our modern-day electrical appliances and equipment all generate within this most dangerous frequency: most laptops and computers generate 12.5 kHz-25 kHz; printers, photocopiers, PlayStations and most electronic equipment generate 10 kHz-100 kHz.

Virtually all of today's modern appliances and energy-efficient electronic devices are drawing their needs within this frequency, creating distortion inside a building's electrical system, thus creating dirty electricity. These include:

- computers
- fax machines
- printers
- photocopiers
- TVs
- entertainment units

- power tools
- variable-speed motors
- energy-efficient appliances
- energy-efficient lighting
- fluorescent lighting
- dimmer switches
- medical equipment

Culprits also include:

- power lines that are loose or in contact with trees
- mobile phone masts, broadcast masts (if not properly filtered)

For example, a plasma TV sends this harmful energy outwards, into the room and into the bodies of the people in it. High measurements of magnetic EMFs have long been of concern with all things electrical, but normally the measurements drop off quickly from the source. These transient EMFs can extend further and when people are surrounded by other electrical equipment in the room, this field is more concentrated.

The increasing use of computers and other electrical devices creates this harmful current. The wiring in our buildings acts as antennae for the current, silently assaulting those who work, live and sleep in the buildings. The wires that deliver electricity everywhere have effectively become a conduit for this harmful energy. We are surrounded by these fields, which now exist on all electrical wiring. These bursts of electromagnetic radiation pack a big burst of energy into a short period of time.

MEASURING DIRTY ELECTRICITY

These fields are particularly harmful because it is now known that this electromagnetic energy penetrates the human body at 1.7 kHz. Martin Graham, emeritus professor of electrical engineering at the University of California, Berkeley and Dave

Stetzer, president of Stetzer Electric Wisconsin, U.S., have designed a meter to measure the actual amount of harmful electrical pollution. The STETZERiZER microsurge meter measures the energy associated with dirty electricity in GS (Graham Stetzer) units, with a range up to 1999 GS units. Any measurement over 1999 GS units - over the scale - displays the numeral '1' on the screen.

Higher cancer incidences in schools and workplaces are more obvious as apart from the higher concentration of people in these buildings, dirty electricity has been found to be especially prevalent in environments with concentrated fluorescent lights and computers. Milham and Morgan used the STETZERiZER microsurge meter (referred to as the GS microsurge meter in the study) for the La Quinta Middle School study. Twenty-five percent of all rooms at this school measured over the scale.

The use of this meter in the cancer cluster at La Quinta Middle School brought further validation on the dangers of exposure to dirty electricity, providing critical information that must be incorporated into our daily lives.

What is important is that dirty electricity showed a positive correlation to cancer incidence at this school:

- Exposure of 1000 GS unit-years increased a teacher's cancer risk by 13 percent.
- Working in a room with a GS overload of more than 2000 GS units for one year increased a teacher's cancer risk by 26 percent.*
- A single year of employment at this school increased a teacher's cancer risk by 21 percent.

* To put 26 percent into perspective, those with the BRCA1 and BRCA2 susceptibility genes are considered to be in the highest risk category for breast cancer. In women, mutations in these genes confer a 40-70 percent risk of breast cancer over the course of their lives. Twenty-six percent over one year is therefore extremely high, even without the addition of further years.

With the teachers being exposed to such high GS units when no more than 30 GS units is recommended emphasises the importance of cleaning up our electrical environments. There is no safe level of exposure. Readings of over 50 GS units (industrial) are considered unacceptable in the Republic of Kazakhstan.

Graham and Stetzer have provided a solution with the STETZERiZER filter. The compact STETZERiZER (GS) filter was designed to remove this harmful electrical pollution. The filters start working at around 1.7 kHz with optimum filtering capacity in a frequency range weapons experts have identified should be protected. The filter simply plugs into an electrical outlet or power strip and is most effective when placed close to the appliance generating the dirty electricity.

The increased prevalence of this radio-frequency current—dirty electricity—has coincided with an alarming increase in the following health disorders:

- Asthma
- Attention-deficit/hyperactivity disorder (ADHD)
- Multiple sclerosis
- Chronic fatigue syndrome
- Fibromyalgia

CANADIAN STUDY

Associate professor Dr Magda Havas of Environmental and Resource Studies, Trent University, Ontario, Canada is one of the leading experts in dirty electricity research and her studies with Dave Stetzer are increasingly reporting that dirty electricity is:

- interfering with education in schools and contributing to behavioural problems among students[10]
- exacerbating symptoms for those suffering from tinnitus and multiple sclerosis
- contributing to electrohypersensitivity (sensitivity to electromagnetic radiation), the most widely reported

symptoms being fatigue and mental impairment (poor memory, reduced concentration and lowered clarity of thought); complaints also include severe headaches, altered sleep patterns, blurred vision, and skin rashes and pain.

RESULTS OF USING FILTERS

The use of the STETZERiZER filters has seen dramatic results. Individuals with multiple sclerosis have had their symptoms *diminish*, reporting better balance and fewer tremors. Those requiring a cane walked unassisted within a few days to weeks after the filters were installed in their home. Dramatic results have been felt only hours after installation.

Fewer and less severe headaches, more energy and less absenteeism are reported in schools that have installed these filters. Improved behaviour associated with ADHD in students has also been reported. The most impressive result in the schools has been regarding students with asthma. After the filters were installed in one Wisconsin school, of the thirty-seven students who had previously used inhalers on a daily basis only three required inhalers, and then for exercise-induced asthma only. After another school in the United States, this one with sick building syndrome, installed filters a lawsuit initiated by the teachers' union was dropped.

Electronic failures, which can be costly, have also been eliminated. Guy Leavitt, superintendent of Blair-Taylor School District in Wisconsin states:

> We did have a number of electronic failures in the district prior to installing the [GS] filters. Since installing them, we have eliminated nearly all of these types of failures. Over the three-year period we may have saved in the range of $40,000.[11]

The groundbreaking study at La Quinta Middle School, one of the most significant of our times, strongly indicates the need for the mandatory measuring and filtering of all buildings world-wide.

> **'Dirty electricity is adversely affecting the lives of millions of people.'**
>
> -Dr Magda Havas and Dave Stetzer, presenting at the WHO conference on electrical hypersensitivity, Prague 2004

> **'Filtration of dirty electricity reduced levels to under 30 GS units, and the patient noticed a dramatic and consistent improvement in sleep patterns within 1 week.'**
>
> -Dr Genuis, Faculty of Medicine, University of Alberta, Edmonton, Canada, *Journal of the Royal Institute of the Royal Institute of Public Health*, 2007

> **'Three days after 16 GS filters were placed in his home his symptoms began to disappear ... He assumed his body was recovering spontaneously but he had been diagnosed with progressive MS and not relapsing/remitting MS, so spontaneous recovery was unlikely in his case.'**
>
> —Dr Magda Havas, *Electromagnetic Biology and Medicine* 25:259, 2007

> **'One teacher in the Wisconsin school that was filtered had been diagnosed with multiple sclerosis (MS). She was extremely tired, had double vision, had cognitive difficulties and could not remember the names of the students in her 4th grade class. Her health would improve during the summer but her symptoms returned in September. She assumed her problems were mold-related but her symptoms did not improve after the mold was removed from the school. Once the school was filtered her symptoms disappeared.'**
>
> —Dr Magda Havas, *Electromagnetic Biology and Medicine* 25:259, 2007

STEVE'S STORY

Multiple Sclerosis to Remission?

Imagine waking up one morning to find you are a victim of multiple sclerosis (MS). Then imagine being transferred to an emergency ward on a drip and being very, very sick.

Pain, headaches, dizziness, depression, inability to focus visually, extreme fatigue—these were just some of the symptoms I had suffered for years. Normal? No. They were the indicators that I had been suffering from the effects of the autoimmune disease MS.

MRI scans were later to reveal myelin sheaf damage and plaques, seen as large lesions in the brain and central nervous system. My digestive system and bowel function broke down and was getting worse.

Would I die like this? I wondered. My mind and my heart became very fearful with the thought of death, as I knew there was little to no chance of recovery from this degenerative disease.

This is my story of how, with the help of STETZERiZER filters, I reversed the supposedly irreversible effects and symptoms of MS.

The story begins with the GS filters and ends with the power of transforming bio-nutrition for the gut (intestinal health) through the biochemical expertise of my friend and colleague, Professor Bill Rock of Sydney, Australia.

I had heard of MS, but really didn't think much about it. I had seen the terrible symptoms and the pain people suffered but I never thought that one day I would be the one dying in a hospital bed in Royal North Shore Hospital.

That was in November 2001. Fortunately I had researched a powerful fruit juice from Tahiti, and as I drank enough of it I was able leave hospital around four weeks later, but I was still very weak and debilitated.

Around January 2006 I heard that the STETZERiZER filters helped reverse the symptoms of MS. I also read peer-reviewed studies and *La Crosse Tribune* articles. I also watched the documentary *Beyond Coincidence*, which detailed what had happened to victims of dirty electricity and sufferers of MS in the United States and Canada once they had installed the filters.

I still did not fully appreciate, and nor did I understand, the connection between electromagnetic fields-RF radiation and MS until I had my apartment tested for microsurges (high-frequency energy) on the 50-Hz AC electrical wiring in the building.

Instead of being less than 50 GS units and at a level considered 'safe' by the Russians, according to the Graham-Stetzer STETZERiZER meter my place was reading 560 GS units! The electrical utility was silently killing me.

According to research in the United States, this type of high GS reading indicates a possible cancer cluster. I had previously been very close to prostate cancer, with elevated PSA readings. I was one sick boy and deteriorating.

Could the answer to my dilemma and possible turnaround of the symptoms of MS come through lowering the high-frequency radiation on the electrical wiring in my apartment? Was I being electrically irradiated by high-frequency, ubiquitous energy from mobile phones, clock radios, electric blankets, TVs and PCs, in addition to the wiring in the building? Was this what was causing me so much grief?

I installed eleven STETZERiZER filters in my apartment in St Leonards, and these brought the readings down to 60–80 GS units. Twenty-four hours later, for the first time in six years, I began to feel almost symptom free. I was walking a little better, I wasn't falling over as much and my appetite picked up. I was also able to drive long distances again.

Later I increased the GS filters to twenty throughout the apartment, and that brought the readings down to 24–35 GS units. The severity of my MS symptoms reduced immediately. It seemed that the lower the GS-unit readings, the better my health was.

In 2008 I had a second MRI scan and my neurologist declared that I was in remission, although not totally cured. His diagnosis was due to the reduced size and prominence of the demylating plaques. This is my latest condition and I am still improving.

I have written medical reports and have had MRI scans for proof of these claims, but better than that, I have a totally new and healthy life thanks to Dave Stetzer and Professor Martin Graham of the University of California

Berkeley.

Thanks to Donna Fisher for letting me share this testimony. I hope it helps people realise there is hope outside Betaferons and other drugs, and that there is a bright future for those suffering from MS, diabetes, cancer and stroke. Your problem may be related to electromagnetic hypersensitivity and you may not know it. My hope and prayer is that you might experience a turnaround as I did.

> **'The connection between exposure to artificial electromagnetic radiation in high and low frequencies and the changing health of diabetics and MS sufferers is an established fact that has been demonstrated beyond doubt in numerous scientific studies.'**
>
> -Dr Magda Havas, *Diabetes and ElectroMagnetic Fields: the evidence*
> Next-up Organization

CHAPTER 4

Diabetes

The number of diabetics worldwide has increased dramatically, as the following figures show:

1985	30 million
1995	135 million
2000	177 million
2008	250 million
2025	300 million (estimated)

The progress of disease is often invisible, yet with diabetes the health effects of dirty electricity can be measured. The STETZERiZER microsurge meter and the STETZERiZER filter show mathematically and scientifically—the hallmark of acceptance—how dirty electricity can alter bodily processes. For instance, it has been shown that entering an electrically dirty room can raise blood sugar levels and leaving that room can lower blood sugar levels.

The meter and filter system is a valuable tool for measuring *mathematically* the lowering of the levels when the filter is installed in the power point. For example, if the reading on the meter is 1700 GS units before the filter is installed, it may read only 1300 GS units after installation. More filters placed in appropriate power points around the building can bring that figure down closer to zero. The following study shows how dirty electricity can be measured *scientifically*. In 2004 Havas and Stetzer presented the following model to the World Health Organization:

Insulin	Week	Dirty electricity GS Units	Blood sugar (mmoles/L)	(units)
With dirty electricity	1	800	9.4	36
With dirty electricity removed	2	13	64	9
% reduction		(98%)	(32%)	(75%)

PPG: ≥7 mmoles/L is considered by the American Diabetes Association to be diabetec
Model: Electrical Pollution Taskforce, Markham, February 2005—Dr Magda Havas
(Authors Note: A new study recently published in the *Journal of the National Cancer Institute*[12] reported that women with higher insulin levels who are overweight had greater odds of developing breast cancer.)

The above model, which shows the difference between an environment with dirty electricity (800 GS units) and one that has been filtered (13 GS units) provides support for two important conclusions:

- Some diabetics may be over-medicating themselves.
- People may be diagnosed with diabetes when they are not diabetic at all.

In mid 2008, Havas labelled environmental diabetes 'type 3' diabetes. This refers to a diabetic whose blood sugar level is also affected by an environmental trigger such as dirty electricity, which increases blood sugar and insulin in type 3 diabetics. Havas' studies have shown that when the dirty electricity is reduced in the home of diabetics, symptoms diminish. Diabetics with electrohypersensitivity (EHS) have higher plasma-glucose levels and require more medication when exposed to dirty electricity.[13]

Other studies have also shown:

- Type 1 diabetics require less insulin.
- Type 2 diabetics have lower levels of plasma glucose in an electrically clean environment.

Havas suggests that dirty electricity may explain why brittle diabetics have difficulty regulating blood sugar. Havas reports that all the diabetics living near relay antennas can easily prove the damaging effects of exposure to artificial HF microwave radiation by observing the spectacular increase in blood sugar levels when they are close to a source of radiation, as can be seen from the reading noted in their personal glycaemia record.

EHS is recognised as a disability—officially, a fully recognised functional impairment—in Sweden and just recently also in Canada. In the United Kingdom it is recognised as a 'condition'. It is recognised by the United States Access Board, an independent federal agency whose primary mission is accessibility for people with disabilities, and in September 2008 the European Parliament recognised the emergence of EHS.

> '**According to Philips and Philips (2006) 3% of the population has electromagnetic hypersensitivity (EHS) and 35% have symptoms of EHS. If these percentages apply to diabetics then as many as 5–60 million diabetics worldwide may be responding to the poor power quality in their environment …**'
>
> —Dr Magda Havas, *Electromagnetic Biology and Medicine* 25:259, 2007

'GS filters may be effective for improving other medical conditions such as hyperlipidemia and hypercholesterolemia. We have seen the subject's blood consistency change.'

—Study at the Natural Clinic, Yoyogi, Tokyo. Preventive Healthcare, Sugimoto 2006

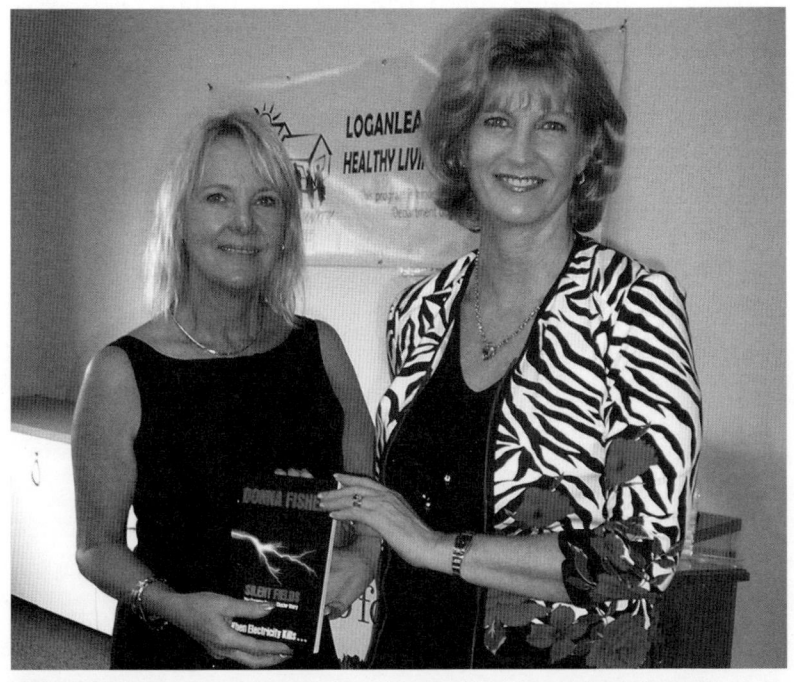

THE FIRST STEP: Pam Parker, mayor of Logan City, Queensland, Australia congratulating the author on the success of her first book *Silent Fields*.

CHAPTER 5

Dirty Electricity and Breast Cancer

Since the 1970s there has been an 80 percent rise in breast cancer cases in the United Kingdom.[14] Between 1973 and 1998 breast cancer rates in the United States increased by more than 40 percent.[15] The use of computers—and the accompanying presence of dirty electricity—has also increased dramatically since the 1970s. Research is continuing into the prevalence of different chemicals as another environmental assault, but, as discussed previously, exposure to EMFs has been shown to enhance the damage from other toxic agents.

The area where the most research has been conducted is that in which our electrical appliances and equipment generate. This is then put back onto the electrical wiring and the power grid: a widely used tower puts out 16.6 kHz, another widely used computer 12.5 kHz, and a widely used laptop computer 25 kHz. Stetzer reports that any energy above 1.7 kHz dissipates internally into the human body.

Stetzer has reported that when a person is working at their computer, the current travels along the muscle tissue and up their arms until it reaches the shoulders. It follows the muscles, which spread out and go in several different directions at the chest before reaching the legs and ultimately the floor. While this current is in the chest muscles, the breast is exposed to the highly dangerous current. It is known beyond doubt that breast tissue is the most sensitive tissue in the body. The fields are amplified and concentrated even more if a woman wears an underwire bra: the current/energy becomes more concentrated in this area due to the wire.

It does not take much current to do some damage at the cellular level. The immune system can no longer repair the damage that the fields cause when the exposure is more than three hours. For younger people and those not in prime health, this is a worst-case scenario.

A wise precaution may be to use a laptop in battery mode only, and have a break while it is charging. And despite its name, placing a laptop on one's lap is not recommended.

COMPUTERS AND CHILDREN

Vladimir Kozlovsky, highly respected professor of medicine and science and deputy director BSE of Infracos-Ecos, Almaty, Kazakhstan compiled a list of norms that need to be in place to limit children's exposure to computers based on their age.[16] He suggested that:

- children younger than seven years be exposed for no more than five minutes
- primary school children be exposed for no more than ten minutes
- fifth grade and older children be limited to thirty minutes per day
- teenagers older than sixteen years limit their computer exposure to less than three hours daily
- pregnant women should not be exposed to computers at all.[17]

COMPUTERS AND THE ELDERLY

In Israel a study was conducted on breast cancer rates in elderly women comparing an earlier period (1978–1990) with a more recent period (1991–2003).[18] The later years were characterised by a much more extensive use of personal computers (more than three hours a day), mobile phones, TV sets and other household electrical appliances than the earlier time period. Available medical records were used that extended over a period of twenty-six years and involved the analysis of more than 200,000 samples.

Among the elderly women who developed breast cancer in the first time frame, 20 percent were regularly exposed to power-frequency fields. But in the more modern period 51 percent were so exposed, mainly through the use of personal computers. The authors concluded that there was 'a statistically significant influence of electromagnetic fields on the formation of all observed epithelial mammary tumours in the second group'. This represented a more than twofold increase, which was considered highly significant.

AREAS OF RISK

Manufacturers of computers are now obliged to limit the magnetic-field measurements emanating from the devices, yet the distance from dirty electricity is of greater concern. Just as baby monitors can blanket a whole house with radio frequency, the dangerous frequencies from computers can blanket the entire room in call centres and workplaces that have areas of concentrated electronic equipment. Call centres could well be a breeding ground for higher incidences of breast cancers.

Stetzer advises that this higher-frequency field is also concentrated in the chairs we sit on when working at computers, as the chair creates another field that poses a risk for the groin area. This is an area of great concern and could be a significant factor explaining why infertility, miscarriage, birth defects, autism, altered sperm quality and quantity, cervical cancer, ovarian cancer and prostate cancers are so prevalent today.

What is also of concern is that these invisible and silent fields are constantly travelling through our bodies, and not only when we are sitting at the computer. They are also riding on the wiring through the walls in our workplaces, schools, hospitals and homes. This insidious and ubiquitous danger is slowly eroding our health, and particularly our breast health.

Traditionally breast cancer was a disease almost exclusively of postmenopausal women but we are now witnessing women in their twenties and thirties being diagnosed. It follows that the younger the female who is exposed to dirty electricity, the greater her risk of breast cancer. The impact of dirty electricity on causation of breast cancer at such an early age is enormous.

Young children, another vulnerable demographic group, are often in front of computers for a large part of their day at schools and universities and they continue to be exposed to computers and other types of electrical equipment into the night.

Dirty electricity, referred to as 'dirty power' by the music industry, is a well-known menace as it can damage sensitive electrical equipment. Singers with microphones at breast level can also be exposed to dirty electricity.

Any exposure of artificially created radiation to the breast should be minimised, particularly for those women with silent carrier genes—or mutations of certain genes—whose sensitivity to the effects of breast carcinogens should be considered. Being born with the silent carrier genes does not cause breast cancer: it increases risk. We must address the causes: the environmental assaults that have increased a woman's lifetime risk of breast cancer so dramatically, from 1:22 in the 1940s to 1:7 in 2004 (US statistics).

Our history has shown that breast tissue is most sensitive to the artificial electromagnetic radiation that we have created, which is known as ionising radiation. It is known beyond doubt that the dropping of the atomic bombs on Nagasaki and Hiroshima caused a dramatic rise in breast cancer incidence in survivors. The rates of breast cancer were highest among females younger than twenty years. A significant association was also reported regarding the incidence of male breast cancer.

It is becoming apparent that we must all be diligently conscious of any form of artificial radiation, and women especially should consider the sensitivity of breast tissue.

THE MANY FORMS OF RADIATION

The following points illustrate the importance of understanding the different types of artificial radiation we are exposed to:

- Ionising radiation includes gamma rays from nuclear bombs, X-rays, CT scans and mammograms. Apart from nuclear fallout, exposure to this form of radiation is by choice.
- Non-ionising radiation includes ELF EMF from electrical wiring, transient EMF from dirty electricity, and RF EMF from communication and wireless sources. Exposure to this form of radiation is on unsuspecting recipients.

Being exposed to high measurements of ELF EMF and transient EMF, and also the radiation from mammograms, chest X-rays and CT scans, could indeed be a potent stimulus for breast cancer growth. With awareness we can and *must* control our exposure.

It is not uncommon for a new technology that is heralded as the best invention of its time to later be recognised as producing undesirable effects. Artificially created radiation is no exception to this. The use of X-rays (including mammograms), once believed to be harmless, is now monitored. Precautions are now in place when X-rays are taken, for both the patient and the operator. The amount of radiation a woman is exposed to in a mammogram is now drastically reduced: down from an average 2 rads in 1976 to 0.2 rads today, one-tenth the original amount. As stated in more depth in *Silent Fields*, there is wide concern over the use of mammograms, especially in younger women, as the challenge of mammography is its ability to cause as well as detect breast cancer. Even though breast cancer awareness, screening and better treatment methods are available, breast cancer incidence continues to increase.

Leading opponents of mammograms are Dr John W Gofman (PhD), who reported that past exposure to ionising radiation—primarily medical X-rays—is responsible for approximately 75 percent of the breast cancer problem in the United States;[19] and Dr Samuel Epstein, chairman of the Cancer Prevention Coalition and professor emeritus of environmental and occupational medicine, University of Illinois School of Public Health, Chicago.

A recently published article in the *British Medical Journal*, 'Breast Screening: The Facts—Or Maybe Not' by Peter Gotzsche and colleagues from the Nordic Cochrane Centre, found women are given one-sided information on screening. The article stated that the leaflet women are given doesn't provide adequate information on the risks of screening for mammograms.

Further to this, Professor Michael Baum, emeritus professor of surgery at University College, London, wrote a letter signed by twenty-two others—representing public health, oncology, GPs, epidemiology and patients—to *The Times* criticising the information that is given to women who are invited to attend National Health Service (NHS) breast cancer screening.[20] The letter says that women in the United Kingdom are not given enough information about the potential harms associated with breast cancer screening, and that for every 2,000 women screened one will benefit (by having her life saved), but ten will have unnecessary treatment, and a further 200 will suffer the worry of being falsely diagnosed with cancer. However, as the letter acknowledges, there is debate about the numbers. Professor Julietta Patnick, director of the NHS cancer screening programmes, countered that this number is closer to an estimated four or five lives saved and four or five women being unnecessarily treated.

Dr Paul Pharoah, a Cancer Research UK researcher at the University of Cambridge, said it was 'imperative' that NHS breast-screening leaflets were rewritten. The leaflets are currently undergoing review.

As the move away from irradiating women's breasts continues, revolutionary technologies—mammography technology is over forty years old—are becoming available.

NEW TECHNOLOGY FOR BREAST CANCER DETECTION

Professor Michael Baum, who was one of the original champions of mammography in the United Kingdom through the NHS, is now on public record as saying he erred. Professor Baum and his colleague Dr Jayant Vaidya are currently using the SureTouch Visual Mapping System[21] and are quickly becoming advocates of its use. This system, often termed a pre-mammogram test, is marketed as non-invasive treatment. It claims to be:

- radiation free
- ultrasound free
- painfree
- not confused by dense breast tissue.

Of immense importance are two-year clinical trials held in the United States and funded by the National Institute of Health (NIH) that showed this system to be more than 94 percent accurate in recognising malignant tumours in both dense and fatty tissue. The results were published in the *American Journal of Surgery*.[22]

Ian McDougall (associate professor) of the Skin Cancer Specialist Centre, Southport, Australia states that from a clinical perspective, SureTouch is unique because it can detect lumps through all areas of the outer aspects of the breast. The system supplies data on the lesion, including estimated size, shape, hardness and location.

> Research indicates that breast cancer arises for four primary reasons: Genetic mutation, altered gene expression, altered cell interaction, or from exposure to agents that alter the body's natural production of estrogen and other hormones.[23]

The progressive Breast Cancer Fund in the United States supports the BioInitiative Report,[24] a scientific review of over two thousand studies. The report stated that the scientific evidence is sufficient to warrant regulatory action for ELF EMF, and is substantial enough to warrant preventative action for RF EMF. Transient EMF (dirty electricity) has characteristics of its own and also has characteristics of both ELF EMF and RF EMF. Many overlapping exposures occur between ELF EMF, transient EMF and RF EMF in our daily lives. Surely there should be a proactive and wise response at a social and government level because of this recently discovered information on dirty electricity. Exposure to toxic agents while in the womb is now considered to be a seed for the development of breast cancer later in life.

Andrew Goldsworthy, honorary lecturer at Imperial College, London, has commented:

> The overall conclusion is that the genetic damage from exposure to electromagnetic radiation can have an almost immediate effect on fertility, but damage to the offspring may take several generations to show up. If we do nothing to limit our exposure to electromagnetic radiation, we can anticipate a slow decline in the viability of the human genome

for many generations to come. It is ironic that having only just discovered the human genome, we have already set about systematically destroying it.

The risk of developing breast cancer is about five times higher in industrialised nations than it is in developing countries, which do not have a prevalence of electricity. It is known that breast cancer occurs more frequently in women who live in more affluent areas; a more comfortable lifestyle usually entails computers and more electrical appliances that contribute to dirty electricity. Until we clean our electrical environments appropriately, we will see the incidence of breast cancer continue to rise, and especially continue to rise in younger females.

As the risk of a female developing breast cancer is very high, what is of critical importance is prevention. This public health issue is so serious that it must be dealt with immediately. It

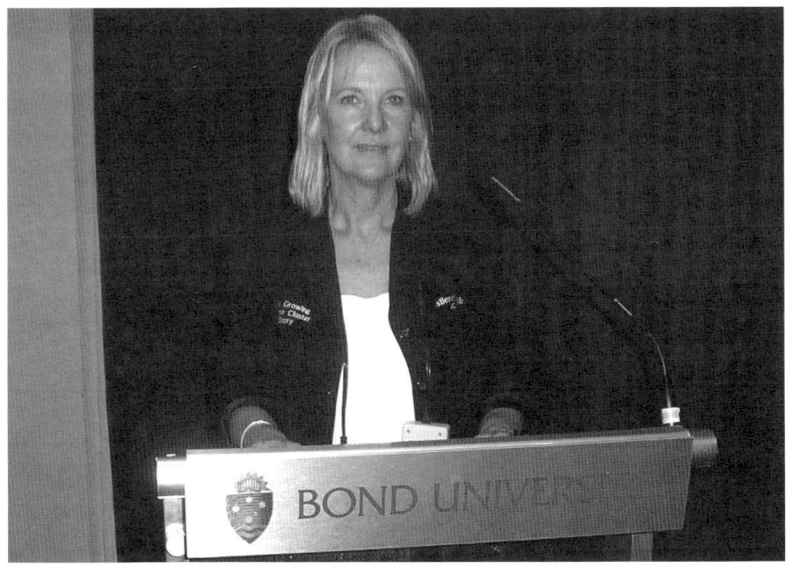

VITAL MESSAGE: The author at Bond University in Australia on why dirty electricity is taking away our breasts.

is a matter of urgency to ensure that we all understand that sitting at a computer for more than three hours, where the environment is not filtered to remove this higher-frequency field, is unacceptable.

Because of this research, in a world that wants to lessen or at best eliminate breast cancer, zero exposure to artificial electromagnetic radiation would be, at the very least, a sensible, intelligent and wise decision. Dirty electricity is the missing link giving further understanding to the dramatic increase in breast cancer statistics.

> **'Successfully preventing breast cancer is one of the greatest challenges faced by science, with benefits to humanity that will one day rank with achievements in exploration of space.'**
>
> —Cedric Garland DPH, epidemiologist and adjunct professor, Department of Family and Preventive Medicine, Cancer Prevention and Control Program, University of California.

CHAPTER 6

The Wireless Revolution

While my first book *Silent Fields* discussed in depth the magnetic field (50/60 Hz) component of electricity, this book focuses more on the higher-frequency field (1–100 kHz). The late Neil Cherry, associate professor at Lincoln University, New Zealand, contended that all radiation across the non-ionising electromagnetic spectrum has contributed to the rise in many cancers, particularly breast cancer, brain tumours and leukaemia. This part of the electromagnetic spectrum includes RF EMF (up to 300 GHz), which our wireless technologies utilise.

Any communication device that is not attached to the wall by a wire is emitting radiation. For example:

- The base units of DECT cordless phones are always radiating, even when no one is using the phone. (Cordless analogue-model base units emit radiation only when the phone is active.)
- A mobile phone that is on but not in use is also radiating. (The mobile is transmitting at maximum power when you connect or disconnect a call, when it is ringing or sending a text message, and when it is being switched on or off.)
- Mobile phone towers are always radiating.
- Wireless networks for computers radiate.

- Wireless microphones to help the hearing-impaired radiate.
- Wireless baby monitors.

Radio-frequency radiation (RF EMF) from wireless technology that flows through the air can be easily received and carried by the electrical wiring network in our buildings. This creates additional dirty electricity, and because this electrical wiring network acts continuously as an antenna, our exposure to this radiation is thus increased.

Mobile phone masts and broadcast masts, if not properly filtered, are also a potent source of dirty electricity that is transferred through the electrical grid into surrounding buildings and houses.

Health effects related to this area of EMFs have been accumulating for decades. In the 1950s and 1960s, workers who built, tested and repaired radar equipment came down with what was later termed 'radiowave sickness', which caused the Russians to study this extensively. During the Cold War the Russian government was accused of bombarding the United States Embassy in Moscow with microwave radiation. The American ambassador became ill and was diagnosed with leukaemia. His replacement also became ill and was diagnosed with leukaemia. Other embassy staff members became ill and had reproductive problems.

When official studies showed the Vatican that radiation levels exceeded the levels set by Italian law, the Vatican authorities claimed the site was sovereign territory and therefore they were not obliged to comply, even though medical reports showed that the incidence of childhood leukaemia in the two-kilometre radius of the Vatican radio site was six times the national average, and the rate of tumours in adults was well beyond the norm.

THE LINK TO MENTAL ILLNESS

In 1974 United States Army researchers reported that low-level microwave radiation—such as that used by mobile phones—might alter the functioning of the blood/brain barrier (BBB).

Swedish scientists repeated this warning in 1992, and also suggested a potential link with Alzheimer's and other neurological diseases.

Swedish neurosurgeon Dr Leif Salford, who has been researching for twenty years, has publicly warned that a whole generation of teenagers using mobile phones may suffer from mental deficiencies or Alzheimer's disease by the time they reach middle age.

Dr Olle Johansson, a neuroscientist at the famous Karolinksa Institute in Stockholm, reports that when second-generation, 1800-MHz mobile phones were introduced into Sweden in 1997 a significant and permanent worsening of the public health began precisely at that time. After a decade-long decline, the number of Swedish workers on sick leave began to rise in late 1997 and more than doubled during the next five years.

During the same period of time, sales of antidepressant drugs also doubled. The number of traffic accidents, after declining for years, began to climb again in 1997. The number of deaths from Alzheimer's disease, after declining for several years, rose sharply in 1999 and had nearly *doubled* by 2001.[25]

INTERNATIONAL ACTION

In their article 'Cancer Trends During the 20th Century',[26] Örjan Hallberg and Olle Johansson (associate professor) reported that in the United States, Sweden and dozens of other countries, mortality rates for skin melanoma, and bladder, prostate, colon, breast and lung cancers closely paralleled the degree of public exposure to radiowaves during the past hundred years. When radio broadcasting increased in a given location, so did those forms of cancer; when it decreased, so did those forms of cancer.[27]

Johansson, along with Brian Stein and Liz Lynne (MP), colleagues of Eileen O'Connor of the UK Radiation Research Trust, recently visited residents living in a cancer cluster around a base station in Kingswinford, UK. Fourteen people in this location have died of cancer, and a further twenty people in the area have been diagnosed with the disease.[28]

The BioInitiative Report stated that the scientific evidence is substantial enough to warrant preventative action for RF EMF. The report concludes that plausible biological mechanisms have already been identified that can reasonably account for most biological effects of exposure to RF EMF at low-intensity levels.

Since the release of the BioInitiative Report in August 2007, moves to lessen exposure to the explosion of wireless technologies is snowballing. The European Parliament demanded in its resolution on 4 September 2008 that the allowable levels for electromagnetic radiation be considerably reduced with regard to public health.

In December 2008 in Valance, France, both the mayor and the opposition agreed—in a political rarity—to mobile phone masts not being erected within one hundred metres of creches and schools. The mayor of Valance, Michele Rivasi, explained:

> First of all because of the scientific BioInitiative Report, which proves the dangers of electromagnetic fields, especially on the nervous system. Number two: a resolution passed by the European Parliament demanding the reduction of permitted radiation levels. Three, the principle of precaution.

Giving legal recognition to the risks posed to human health by mobile phone masts, a legal precedent was established when the Versailles Court of Appeal ordered the dismantling of an antenna mast in Tassin la Demi-Lune in the Rhone. All relay antennae of that particular telecommunications company are now under suspended sentence. A September 2008 judgement stated:

> To expose one's neighbour against his will to a certain risk, and not a hypothetical one as the defence has claimed, constitutes in itself a public nuisance. Its egregious character is due to the fact that it has a bearing on human health. If this risk were to materialise in significant health problems, this would constitute a different type of offence deserving a more severe sentence, in accordance with the gravity of the problems.[29]

In March 2009 a judge in Angers Tribunal de Grande Instance (District Court) prevented the Orange phone company installing a mobile phone antenna in the bell tower of a church next to a school.

In February 2009 the Tribunal de Grande Instance (District Court) of Carpentras ordered, on the grounds of potential health risks and nuisance to one's neighbour, the demolition of a relay telephone mast, with a penalty of 400 euros per day of delay after the fourth month of the announcement of the judgement.[30]

Moves by other countries since the release of the BioInitiative Report include:

- France: The National Library of France dismantled wireless following the decision by the mayor of Paris to turn off WiFi networks in six French libraries.
- Salzburg: The Salzburg Public Health Department issued a letter to all schools and kindergartens recommending avoidance of wireless technologies.
- Germany: Actively advised on how to reduce personal exposure: warning of 'electrosmog' from baby monitors to electric blankets; advised against wireless; recommended cabled connections and the use of landlines instead

of mobiles (including the Frankfurt Local Education Authority and German Teachers Union).
- Belgium: The minister responsible for consumer protection would not authorise the marketing of mobile phones intended for children due to the cumulative risks of radiation.
- Austria: The Austrian Medical Association published a recommendation to use cables instead of WiFi.
- Canada: Lakehead University restricted the use of WiFi.
- Taiwan: Hundreds of towers have been dismantled.
- Finland: The Radiation and Nuclear Safety Authority (STUK) recommended restricting children's use of mobile phones.
- Israel: Restricted antennae on residential buildings and cautioned that the specific microwave frequency at which mobile phones broadcast utilises the human head as an antenna and the brain tissue as a radio receiver.
- Australia: Professor Bruce Armstrong recommended that the ALARA principle be implemented, especially when it comes to children and mobile phones.
- United Kingdom: The chief of a 38,000-strong teachers union called for WiFi in schools to be suspended due to reports linking it to loss of concentration, fatigue, reduced memory and headaches, and the fear of its impact on the developing nervous systems of children.
- United Kingdom: Sir William Stewart, the UK government's chief adviser on mobile phone safety, called for a ban on erecting phone masts near schools, and warned of the risks of allowing children, whose thin skulls can more easily be penetrated by radiation, to use mobile phones.
- Russia: Recommendations listed in the Sanitary Rules of the Ministry of Health insisted that children under eighteen years should not use mobile phones.

In November 2008, Liechtenstein became the first country to mandate lower emission standards—by ten times—to go into effect in 2013. The emissions from outdoor antennae used by mobile phones, radar, TV and FM broadcasting, and wireless internet are to be 0.1 $\mu W/cm^2$ or 0.614 V/m, which is the limit for the city of Salzburg and is also recommended in the BioInitiative Report.

Of immense importance, on 1 April 2009 the European Parliament passed the European Parliament EMF Resolution: 'Health concerns associated with electromagnetic fields.'[31]

The progressive Breast Cancer Fund in the United States supported the findings of the BioInitiative Report, namely that the scientific evidence is substantial enough to warrant preventative actions for RF EMF. The Breast Cancer Fund also stated that, based on the scientific evidence set forth in the BioInitiative Report and a growing body of additional research, exposure limits for electromagnetic radiation should be set at the federal level. The European Environmental Agency also supported the BioInitiative Report.

The e-book *Public Health SOS: The Shadow Side of the Wireless Revolution* provides an in-depth explanation of this emerging health issue and answers more than one hundred frequently asked questions.[32]

Arthur Firstenberg reported in *The Largest Biological Experiment Ever* that two minutes on a mobile phone disrupts the BBB, two hours on a mobile phone causes permanent brain damage, and secondhand radiation may be almost as bad.[33]

CHILD PROTECTION IN RUSSIA

The following report on the dangers of children using mobile phones comes from the Russian National Committee on Non-Ionising Radiation Protection, Moscow, Russia:

> For the first time in history, we face a situation where most

children and teenagers in the world are continuously exposed to the potentially adverse effects of electromagnetic fields (EMF) from mobile phones.

An electromagnetic field is an important biotropic factor, affecting not just human health in general but also the processes of the higher nervous activity, including behaviour and thinking. Radiation directly affects the human brain when people use mobile phones.

Despite the recommendations listed in the Sanitary Rules of the Ministry of Health, which insist that persons under 18 years should not use mobile phones ... children and teenagers became the target group for the marketing of mobile communications.

The current safety standards for exposure to microwaves from mobile phones have been developed for adults and don't consider the characteristic features of children's organisms. The WHO considers the protection of children's health from the possible negative influence of EMF from mobile phones as the highest priority. This problem has also been confirmed by the Scientific Committee of the European Commission, by national authorities of European and Asian countries, and by participants of international scientific conferences on biological effects of the EMF.

The potential risk for children's health is very high:

- The absorption of electromagnetic energy in a child's head is considerably higher than in an adult's head (children's brains are smaller, have higher conductivity, thinner skull bones, and a smaller distance from the antenna).
- Children's organisms have greater sensitivity to EMF than adults'.
- Children's brain have greater sensitivity to the accumulated adverse effects relating to chronic exposure to EMF.
- EMF affects the formation of the process of the higher

nervous activity.
- Today's children will spend significantly more time using mobile phones than will today's adults.

According to the opinion of the Russian National Committee on Non-Ionizing Radiation Protection, the following health hazards are likely to be faced by children using mobile phones in the immediate future: disruption of memory, decline of attention, diminishing learning and cognitive abilities, increased irritability, sleep problems, increase in sensitivity to stress, increased epileptic readiness.

Expected (possible) remote health risks: brain tumours, tumours of acoustical and vestibular nerves (in the age 25–30 age group), Alzheimer's, 'got dementia', depressive syndrome, and other types of degeneration of the nervous structures of the brain (in the 50–60 age group).

The members of the Russian National Committee on Non-Ionizing Radiation Protection emphasise the urgency of defending children's health from the influence of EMF from mobile communication systems. We appeal to government authorities and to the entire society to pay closest attention to this coming threat and to take adequate measures to prevent negative consequences to future generations' health.

Children using mobile communications are not aware of the risks in subjecting their brains to EMF radiation. We believe that this risk is not much lower than the risk to children's health from tobacco or alcohol. It is our professional obligation not to allow this damage children's health by inactivity.[34]

> 'In the United States now there are seven class action lawsuits active against the cell phone industry, the mobile phone industry. To put that into context, it was one class action that brought down the asbestos industry and it was one class action that put the silicone breast implant industry into bankruptcy. There are seven active class actions.'
>
> —Dr George Carlo, chairman, Science and Public Policy Institute (non profit), USA, 2007[35]

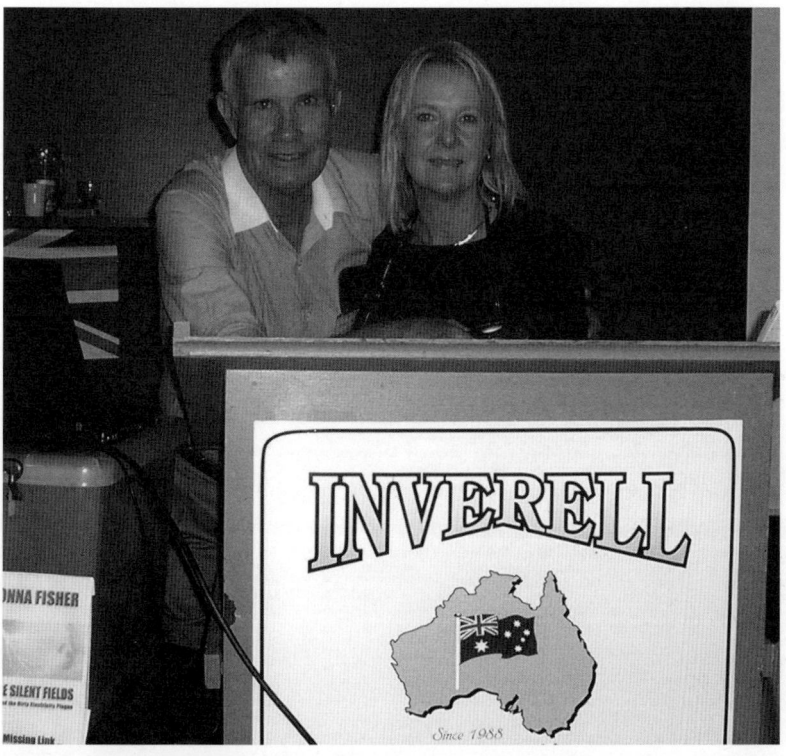

INVERELL FORUM: The thirst for information in simple, easily understood terms is overwhelming.

CHAPTER 7

The Venice Resolution

Over fifty scientists worldwide signed the Benevento Resolution of September 2006, which called for, along with other recommendations:

- the promotion of alternatives to wireless technologies
- limiting the use of mobile and cordless phones and the manufacture of phones that radiated away from the head
- planning communications antennae to minimise human exposure.

Soon after, these scientists took exception to the claim from the wireless communication industry that there was no credible scientific evidence to conclude there was a risk. This resulted in the signing of the Venice Resolution in June 2008, as recent epidemiological evidence is more compelling than ever. Scientists saw this evidence as a further reason to justify precautions being taken to lower exposure standards in accordance with the precautionary principle.

Initiated by the International Commission for Electromagnetic Safety, the Venice Resolution is as follows:

> As stated in the Benvento Resolution of September 2006, we remain concerned about the effects of human exposure to

electromagnetic fields on health. At the Venice Workshop, entitled, 'Foundations of bioelectromagnetics: towards a new rationale for risk assessment and management,' we discussed electro-hypersensitivity, blood/brain barrier changes, learning and behavioural effects, changes in anti-oxidant enzyme activities, DNA damage, biochemical mechanisms of interaction, biological damage and, experimental approaches to validate these effects. As an outcome, we are compelled to confirm the existence of non-thermal effects of electromagnetic fields on living matter, which seem to occur at every level of investigation from molecular to epidemiological.

An urgent task before international researchers is to discover the detailed mechanisms of non-thermal interactions between electromagnetic fields and living matter. A collateral consequence will be the design of new general public and occupational protection standards. We, who are at the forefront of this research, encourage an ethical approach in setting of exposure standards which protect the health of all, including those who are more vulnerable. We recognize the need for research to reveal the critical exposure parameters of effect and risk from exposure to electromagnetic fields.

The non-ionising radiation protection standards recommended by international standards organizations, and supported by the World Health Organization, are inadequate. Existing guidelines are based on results from acute exposure studies and only thermal effects are considered. A world wide application of the Precautionary Principle is required. In addition, new standards should be developed to take various physiological conditions into consideration, e.g., pregnancy, newborns, children, and elderly people.

We take exception to the claim of the wireless communication industry that there is no credible scientific evidence to conclude there a risk. Recent epidemiological evidence is stronger than before, which is a further reason to justify precautions be taken to lower exposure standards in accordance with the

Precautionary Principle.

We recognize the growing public health problem known as electrohypersensitivity; that this adverse health condition can be quite disabling; and, that this condition requires further urgent investigation and recognition.

We strongly advise limited use of cell phones, and other similar devices, by young children and teenagers, and we call upon governments to apply the Precautionary Principle as an interim measure while more biologically relevant standards are developed to protect against, not only the absorption of electromagnetic energy by the head, but also adverse effects of the signals on biochemistry, physiology and electrical biorhythms.

For a full list of the signees of the Venice Resolution, see Appendix E.

> **'This is real evidence that hyperfrequency electromagnetic fields can have geno-toxic effects. And this damaged DNA is always the cause of cancer. We've found these damaging effects on the genes at levels well below the safety limits. That's why we think it's urgent to base our safety limits on the biological effects and not on the thermic ones. They should be based on biology, not on physics.'**
>
> —Professor Franz Adlekofer, coordinator of the Reflex report[36]

CHAPTER 8

Autism

The autistic-child syndrome, first described in 1943, has had an astonishing 6,000 percent increase in recent years, which parallels the staggering increase in these silent and invisible fields. American advocacy groups call autism 'the fastest-growing developmental disability in the United States'. Precautionary measures must now be taken whilst pregnant as the pelvic structure promotes deep RF radiation penetration which can be absorbed by the developing foetus.

Dr Robert Becker cautioned back in 1990 that 'the apparent onset of autism as a clinical condition in the early 1940s does coincide with the marked increase in our usage of electromagnetic energy'. He believed it was vitally important to determine whether autism is the result of exposure to abnormal electromagnetic fields, either during the final stages of foetal life or at the early newborn stage.[37] EMF researcher B Blake Levitt suspects that EMF from Doppler ultrasound may be harming foetuses: autism rates have skyrocketed since the medical profession first began using the technology.

The artificial electromagnetic radiation/electromagnetic fields we have created appear to affect our neurochemistry in far-reaching ways. The younger the person exposed to radiation the more concern there is about biological effects. Dr Cornelia O'Leary, a fellow of the Royal College of Surgeons in England, studied the possible relationship between SIDS and abnormal electromagnetic fields. In the late 1980s she reported that eight such deaths occurred in one weekend (four of these within a single two-hour period) within a radius of seven miles (a little over eleven kilometres) of a top-secret military base where a powerful new radar unit was being tested.[38]

Not many studies of an EMF/autism relationship have been conducted to date. A 2007 groundbreaking scientific study published in the peer-reviewed *Journal of the Australasian College of Nutritional and Environmental Medicine* warned that wireless communication technology may be responsible for the accelerating rise in autism among the world's children.[39] The primary author of the paper is Tamara Mariea, a certified clinical nutritionist and director of Internal Balance Inc, based in Nashville, Tennessee, who specialises in treating autism and who has helped over five hundred autistic children since 2000. Mariea collaborated with Dr George Carlo, expert on the dangers of electromagnetic radiation (EMR) and chairman of the non-profit Science and Public Policy Institute in the United States, the world's largest research program on mobile phone health hazards in the 1990s.

Mariea and Carlo's work revealed the autism-wireless technology connection following a series of tests on autistic children monitored during 2005 and 2006. Carlo stated:

> Although some of the increase in autism can be ascribed to more efficient diagnosis by the medical community, a rise of this magnitude must have a major environmental cause. Our data offer a reasonable mechanistic explanation for a connection between autism and wireless technology ... These findings tie in with other studies showing adverse cell-membrane responses and disruptions of normal cell physiology. The EMR apparently causes the metals to be trapped in cells, slowing clearance and accelerating the onset of symptoms.

AUTISM AND HEAVY METAL

Autism is a disabling neuro-developmental disorder whose cause is not completely understood, but it is known to involve heavy-metal toxicity.[40]

Of particular interest, in Kazakhstan metallurgical industries have a high morbidity rate and many people become invalids. Many exposed workers have had reduced life expectancy, with people often dying by the age of fifty. Workers in the metallurgical industries associated with electrolytic metal extraction are exposed to high EMFs. E Zharkinov, professor of medicine and head of occupational hygiene, Kazakhstan Scientific Center of Hygiene and Epidemiology, reports that the electrical field exposures had a synergistic, negative effect with the simultaneous heavy-metal exposure to make the situation in those industries more hazardous.[41]

We must take heed of Carlo's warnings as Alzheimer's disease may well take over the acknowledged childhood leukaemia risk as a more recent study reports a compelling dose-response relationship. Carlo stated:

> The thing that we have identified here, this mechanism with these children with autism, what is happening in general … is they have the heavy metal build up because of their vaccines. They are exposed to the information-carrying radio waves, the active transport channels close down and heavy metals like mercury get caught inside the cell. The heavy metals disrupt the talking between messenger RNA (Ribonucleic acid) and DNA and you have an environmentally induced genetic change that appears in the daughter cells. This is serious and this is happening. If you do the same exposure scenario in an older person, you have symptoms that look like Alzheimer's disease.[42]

There is already strong evidence that long-term exposure to EMFs is a risk factor for Alzheimer's disease, and the latest study conducted by doctors at Bern University's Institute of Social and Preventative Medicine in Switzerland makes the evidence even stronger. The study found that the risk of developing Alzheimer's increases the longer people live next to electricity pylons: 'Anyone who lives within the immediate vicinity of high-voltage power lines for more than 10 years has a significantly higher risk of developing dementia or Alzheimer's.'[43]

Professor Denis Henshaw of the HH Wills Physics Department of Bristol University stated that the paper was 'like the final piece of a jigsaw. The link between childhood leukaemia and power lines is already accepted by everybody'.

Professor Egger, who headed the study, warns that sleeping next to a radio-operated alarm clock or living beside an electrified railway line present a similar dementia risk, due to proximity of the radiation source and the strength of the electrical charge.

With the different wireless devices, and equipment and communications antennae permeating our environments, everyone in the developed world is surrounded by a proliferation of artificial radio-frequency waves creating an artificial electromagnetic blanket that constantly envelops us. In fact, even if you were to live on a mountaintop without electricity, exposure to communication frequency would be likely. Everyone is exposed to a greater or lesser extent, with vulnerable populations—pregnant women, foetuses, young children—exposed to the same degree as the general population: no unexposed populations exist.

The rollout of the new 3G (third generation) wireless phones—and related, community-wide antenna RF emissions—in the Netherlands caused almost immediate public complaints of illness.[44]

The advent of WiMAX is also of great concern: higher levels of RF are produced at the wireless transmission facilities than for WiFi. At this point in time, in the promotion of alternatives to wireless communications systems the scientists who signed the Benevento Resolution recommend the use of fibre optics and coaxial cables.

The BioInitiative Report concluded that RF EMF exposure can be considered genotoxic—will damage our precious DNA our blueprint for growth and development—under certain conditions of exposure.

BABY MONITORS

Another area of increasing concern is the radiation from wireless baby monitors, something that has concerned scientists for many years. Dr Andrew Goldsworthy, retired lecturer in biology from the Imperial College, London and signee of the Benevento Resolution and the Venice Resolution wrote to Sir William Stewart, chairman of Britain's Health Protection Agency:

Dear Sir William

As I guess you know, there has been considerable press publicity about a possible link between the 6000 percent increase in autism in recent years and the proliferation of mobile telecommunications and Wifi.

With hindsight we might have expected this, since their radiations have non-thermal effects on brain function. As I explained in my article at http://tinyurl.com/2nfujj (which I believe that you read some months ago), pulsed electromagnetic radiation removes structurally-important calcium ions from cell membranes and increases their tendency to leak. When this happens in neurones, it will generate spurious action potentials to create a 'mental fog', which reduces a person's ability to perform complex functions such as driving a car. This is almost certainly the explanation for the four-fold increase in the accident rate when driving a car while using a mobile phone (even when are using a hands-free type).

However, even more serious is that the same mechanism could induce autism in babies. Just after its birth, a child's brain is essentially a blank canvas and it goes through an intense period of learning to become aware of the significance of all its new sensory inputs, e.g. to recognise its mother's face, her expressions and eventually other people and their relationship to him. If these processes are disrupted by spurious action potentials, they may be hindered, not accomplished in the allotted time, and the child may then express all the symptoms of autism.

A useful analogy might be the socialisation of dogs. If puppies do not meet and interact with other dogs within the first four months of their life, they too develop autistic behaviour. They become withdrawn, afraid of other dogs and strangers, and are incapable of normal 'pack' behaviour. Once this four-month window has been passed, the effect seems to be irreversible (i.e. just like autism).

Whether you believe my explanation for the production of spurious action potentials is a matter for personal preference, but the brain is nevertheless an electrical organ and we should not be too surprised if it is affected by extraneous electromagnetic fields, and that the 'blank canvas' of a newborn child's brain may be particularly susceptible.

While these effects might occur in response to the general electromagnetic environment, the use of cordless digital baby alarms may put the child especially at risk due to chronic exposure from a nearby source. Is it possible to get information on any correlation between the use of digital cordless baby alarms and autism and possibly other childhood problems such as cot death? If so, and the results prove positive, it may be necessary to take these devices off the shelves and advise people not to use them.

Yours sincerely
Dr Andrew Goldsworthy[45]

A recent pilot research study has shown higher rates of babies born with autism where the mothers' sleeping locations had high levels of RF electromagnetic radiation.[46]

'There is some anecdotal evidence that autistic children improve if the power quality in their environment is improved.'[47] Filtering the electrical environment can improve the power quality.

In what has been described as a monumental breakthrough, in April 2009 researchers found that DNA changes affecting genes related to early brain development are involved in as many as 15 percent of cases. Hakon Hakonarson of The Children's Hospital of Philadelphia, who led the groundbreaking research, stated:

> Because other researchers have made intriguing suggestions that autism arises from abnormal connections among brain cells during early development, it's very compelling to find evidence that mutations in genes involved in brain interconnections increase a child's risk of autism.

Considering that EMFs have been shown to cause changes in the way DNA works and breaks, the crucial question is: What will be the cost if we continue to expose the highly sensitive brain and body tissue of newborn babies so intimately to artificially created electromagnetic radiation?

'A new scientific truth does not triumph by convincing its opponents and making them see the light, but rather because its opponents eventually die, and a new generation grows up that is familiar with it.'

—Max Planck, winner of Nobel Prize in Physics

A FATHER'S STORY

Autism

In January 2009 we installed fifteen STETZERiZER filters in our home. We were interested to see if they could provide any improvement for our four year old son who suffers from autism. Since installing the filters we have recognised a considerable improvement in our son's behaviour. He is more open to the world around him and we see a lot of progress with his cognitive abilities. A month after we installed the filters he started to read letters and numbers on cars and he completed the alphabet for the first time in his life. Three months later he could speak more words and he expresses his own will (which he did not do before). Nowadays he is also very interested in puzzles.

I am convinced that the filters are not just a pill for my own headaches (I notice that the pain disappears immediately) but they also seem to have allowed my son's brain to commence a repair process.

In my opinion, although the brain of our son still has to repair and develop further, at this rate of improvement we expect to have made up significant lost ground by the end of this year.

J de Hass
The Hague, The Netherlands

CHAPTER 9

Genes versus Environment

Lichtenstein et al concluded from their study of identical twins in 2000 that environmental factors were the initiating event in the majority of cancers.[48] The effects of these artificial EMFs on particular genes and the build-up of defective genes due to the EMFs have already been noticed.

Cancer risk is related to DNA damage; the genes are damaged. Cells with damaged DNA either die or are repaired. If repaired properly, there are no further problems. DNA that is not entirely repaired or not repaired correctly leads to changes in chromosomes and mutations that can precipitate the development of cancer. Critical genetic mutations in one single cell are sufficient to progress to cancer. Inheriting a mutated gene, or having a gene become mutated, increases cancer risk. When the rate of damage to DNA exceeds the rate at which DNA can be repaired, the opportunity is there for cancer to develop.

Life and our health is dependent on the health and function of the different genes that control when and how our cells grow, divide and die, a delicate timing process that is constantly occurring in our bodies. Cancer develops when there is an imbalance between cell growth and cell death. The cell cycle while in the womb and in young children, however, is much quicker. The faster the cells duplicate, the higher the chance that something can go wrong. DNA damage and altered cell function can accelerate tumour development.

Cancer is characterised by cell division that has gone out of control. This is why it is so very important to protect the developing child from any substance that may affect this process, and it is also why women are asked if they are pregnant before they are exposed to X-rays, CT scans and mammograms.

Ionising radiation causes cancer by directly damaging DNA and disrupting normal cellular and intra-cellular processes. It is acknowledged that ionising-radiation damage to genes is cumulative over a lifetime. With regard to non-ionising radiation, EMF research has also shown disruption of normal cellular and intra-cellular processes. Research indicates that the effects are cumulative, and that at the gene level ELF EMF and RF EMF can cause changes in how DNA works.

Earlier research reported that childhood leukaemia could be triggered while in the womb. Leukaemia has presented in the children of women who worked with industrial sewing machines, where exposure to magnetic fields can be very high.[49] Studies (ELF EMF) conducted in the 1980s showed birth defects in the children of exposed male workers,[50] with Becker commenting that the exposure produced abnormalities in the chromosomes of the sperm. (All the more reason to caution against having your mobile phone in your trouser pocket!)

Brain tumours and nervous-system cancers have been reported in children when fathers were exposed to high levels of EMFs.[51] The children and adults of today have already been affected.

Andrew Goldsworthy, honorary lecturer at Imperial College, London comments:

> 'Heavy mobile phone use appears to reduce both the quantity and viability of sperm. The results for the most recent study by Dr Ashok Agarwal and co-workers at the Cleveland Lerner College of Medicine can be seen at http://tinyurl.com/28rm6n.

They found that using a mobile phone for more than four hours a day was associated with a reduction in sperm viability and mobility of around 25 percent. The statistical probability of these results being due to chance errors was one in a thousand. There is every reason to believe that human eggs may be similarly affected, but since they are formed in the embryo before the baby is born, the damage will be done during pregnancy but will not become apparent until the child reaches puberty.'

Just as women are seen to be more at risk of developing breast cancer if they have certain silent carrier genes, men are also. Most cancers—particularly breast and ovarian cancer—associated with BRCA1 and BRCA2 mutations are seen in women, but men with these mutations are also at higher risk for male breast cancer, as well as prostate and pancreatic cancer, and melanoma.

The very latest and groundbreaking research is reporting that people with certain genes or defective genes could be particularly sensitive to the carcinogenic effects of non-ionising EMF/EMR.[52] The XRCC1 gene is one of many known to help repair DNA damage. A defective variant of this gene, 'rs25489' SNP,[53] has been shown to make its carriers more likely to develop breast and prostate cancer, and now leukaemia. Of immense interest, Mexican-Americans are much more likely to carry this SNP, and it has been reported that children in Mexico City have greater exposure to magnetic fields than those in other countries, often more than 6 mG units.[54]

This combination could well explain why statistics compiled by the Centers for Disease Control and Prevention in the United States show that Mexico has one of the highest incidences of leukaemia in the world.[55]

RADIOWAVES AND LUNG CANCER

It is not only due to its vastness that this important health issue will dwarf the cigarette-smoking and asbestos issues combined. These artificial electromagnetic fields have already been shown to enhance the damage of other toxic agents. The missing pieces of the puzzle as to why there is so much cancer started to appear when Örjan Hallberg and Olle Johansson looked at cancer trends during the twentieth century. These fields, which we have created, may well also be the underlying menace in the cigarette-smoking and asbestos crises.[56] The following information is taken from Hallberg and Johansson's article 'Cancer Trends During the 20th Century':

> An automated computer analysis of the age-specific incidence of lung cancer among men in Sweden points at year 1955 as the starting year for a sudden environmental change in Sweden and that this disturbance mainly affects men over sixty years of age. This method of analysis has successfully been applied to study the development of melanoma of skin in Sweden, Norway, Denmark, Finland, and the United States.[57]

What happened in Sweden in 1955? In 1955, FM radio and TV1 was introduced, along with the accompanying artificially created radiowaves. Hallberg and Johansson noticed, relatively shortly after the introduction of FM radio, that people who had been smoking for many years were suddenly presenting with lung cancer. The abrupt increase was not noticed in countries where FM radio had not been rolled out. For instance, Estonia had a steep increase in cancer mortality in 1991, the year that Western FM radio frequencies were allowed and introduced all over the country. In 2002, Hallberg and Johansson found statistically that country by country—and county to county within Sweden—exposure to radiowaves appeared to be *as big a factor in causing lung cancer as cigarette smoking*.[58]

This does not mean we should keep on smoking cigarettes.

This information indicates that we should stop smoking because we are all exposed to EMR and it is exacerbating the damage from the chemical carcinogens in cigarettes.

THE MELANOMA LINK

Also in Sweden, skin melanoma statistics started to explode from 1955–1996, an increase of more than fourteen times than before 1955. A similar steep rise in melanoma mortality was also reported in Queensland, Australia when comparing 1951–1959 with 1964–1967. This increase was related to the introduction of high-power TV broadcasting transmitters. Skin melanoma has also been associated with the expansion of broadcasting networks in Sweden, Norway, Denmark and the United States.

Augustsson and Stierner presented statistics on the location of moles, melanocytes and melanoma on the human body, with the highest to lowest areas in descending order being: chest and back, abdomen and buttocks, lower legs, thighs, arms, head and feet. Hallberg and Johansson believe that the induced currents from RF exposure are largest at these parts of the body, so the mole density should be expected to follow the same pattern.

Of interest, the increase in melanoma that has occurred since the 1950s cannot be adequately explained by environmental exposure to ultraviolet radiation. Extensive research in Sweden recently confirmed that adverse electromagnetic radiation is a determinant in the development of malignant melanoma, an increasingly prevalent cancer that was uncommon until about fifty years ago. Hallberg and Johansson reported a strong association between non-ionising radiation—FM radio, 100 MHz—and the existence of malignant melanoma of the skin.[59]

In their work, Hallberg and Johansson showed how weak the connection is between lung cancer and cigarette consumption in Swedish countries. A number of countries postulated that if lung cancer mortality is normalised to the melanoma of skin mortality in the same countries, a very strong correlation suddenly appears. Lung cancer mortality has a multiple correlation to both cigarette consumption and skin melanoma mortality.

They report that this indicates *a common factor behind the rapidly increasing mortality rates of skin and lung cancer.* A closer look at lung cancer mortality shows a development very similar to skin melanoma. Lung cancer has had an almost identical development to melanoma in Sweden, with a scale factor of ten. Further to this, figures of melanoma and breast cancer incidences from forty countries show an association. They concluded that breast cancer and lung cancer are linked to skin melanoma. The large numbers involved in this analysis exclude the possibility that the results are just a matter of coincidence. Breast and prostate cancers are correlated. People who move from low- to high-incidence countries also increase their chances. Breast, bladder, prostate, lung, colon and cutaneous melanoma cancers are all correlated, with a strong relationship between melanoma and colon cancer, and between lung cancer and bladder cancer.

Hallberg and Johansson concluded that there is a common environmental stress that accelerates several cancer forms, such as colon cancer, lung cancer, breast cancer, bladder cancer and malignant melanoma.

THE WORLD TODAY

Since electricity was first generated—when the possibility of electrocution was regarded as the only hazardous side effect—to our now wireless world, exposure to electromagnetic radiation and the adverse health effects ranging from fatigue to serious disease and cancer have exploded within a brief time window of our history:

1900	Electricity
1920	AM radio
1940	Radar
1950	FM radio, TV
1970	Computers
1980	Mobile phones
2000	WiFi, WiMAX, compact fluorescent lamps (CFLs)

Dirty electricity has characteristics of RF EMF. This higher-frequency field is also in the radiowave part of the electromagnetic spectrum. By operating our computers, PlayStations, fax machines, printers and the like we are creating additional implications for our health.

Due to the dramatic cancer statistics from the fallout of the atomic bombs dropped on Hiroshima and Nagasaki, ionising radiation was the first known cause of cancer. The non-ionising part of the electromagnetic spectrum, treated as harmless by many, is even more of a threat. It has been woven into our whole way of living. We can no longer remain guarded, inactive and silent on the most serious contender and most likely culprit responsible for the staggering increase in ill-health and cancers: constant exposure to the unrestrained use of this artificially created electromagnetic energy.

> '**I have no doubt in my mind that at the present time that the greatest polluting element in the earth's environment is the proliferation of electromagnetic fields. I consider that to be far greater on a global scale than warming ...**'
>
> —Robert O Becker, MD, *The Body Electric: Electromagnetism and the Foundation of Life*, 1998; *Cross Currents: The Perils of Electropollution: The Promise of Electromedicine*, 1990

RADIOWAVE SICKNESS

The medical term 'radiowave sickness' was first used by Russian doctors to describe an occupational illness developed by large numbers of workers exposed to microwave or radio frequency radiation. Studies date back to 1960. Electrohypersensitivity (EHS) is a newer term and radio frequency sickness is also used. Symptoms of exposure to radio-frequency radiation/radiowave sickness/EHS, which was first documented among radar workers during the Second World War, include:[60]

- Neurological: headaches, dizziness, nausea, difficulty concentrating, memory loss, irritability, depression, anxiety, insomnia, fatigue, weakness, tremors, muscle spasms, numbness, tingling, altered reflexes, muscle and joint pain, leg/foot pain, 'flu-like' symptoms, fever. More severe reactions can include seizures, paralysis, psychosis and stroke.
- Cardiac: palpitations, arrhythmias, pain or pressure in the chest, low or high blood pressure, slow or fast heart rate, shortness of breath.
- Respiratory: sinusitis, bronchitis, pneumonia, asthma.
- Dermatological: skin rash, itching, burning, facial flushing.
- Ophthalmologic: pain or burning in the eyes,

pressure in/behind the eyes, deteriorating vision, floaters, cataracts.
- Others: digestive problems; abdominal pain; enlarged thyroid, testicular/ovarian pain; dryness of lips, tongue, mouth, eyes; great thirst; dehydration; nosebleeds; internal bleeding; altered sugar metabolism; immune abnormalities; redistribution of metals within the body; hair loss; pain in the teeth; deteriorating fillings; impaired sense of smell; ringing in the ears.

Common sources of radiowaves (wired and wireless) include:[61]

- Outdoors: broadcast and mobile phone antennae, radar, mobile phones, pagers, two-way radios.
- Indoors: cordless telephones and their base units, wireless computers and their base units, wired computers, televisions, microwave ovens, dimmer switches, security systems, remote controls, fax machines, answering machines, assistive listening systems and devices for the hearing impaired, wireless microphones, variable-speed motors, transformers, cordless baby monitors, electric utility smart meters, signal-broadcasting smoke alarms, some electronic games.
- Vehicles: CB radios, ignition systems, mobile radar units.

CHAPTER 10

Cancer Treatment Using Radiowaves

Although a lot is known about cancer, the mechanism of cancer in general is not known. Scientists though have been aware since the earlier part of the twentieth century that electrical energy can target cancer cells: in an intruiging case in Cork, Ireland, a woman was struck by lightning and her breast cancer went away.

My first book, *Silent Fields*, pointed out the paradox of these fields being harmful as well as being a possible method of healing. At the time of writing, compelling research has come to light regarding the efficacy of precision-focused RF energy. An earlier review was conducted for all the work done up to 1999 but the treatment methods and technology are constantly being improved.

The three modalities that are currently used for cancer treatment are surgery, radiation (ionising) and chemotherapy. As the overall contribution of chemotherapy (curative and adjuvant cytotoxic) to 5-year survival in adults was estimated to be 2.3 percent in Australia and 2.1 percent in the United States,[62] a fourth modality (the scientific term is hyperthermia) using ultra-high-frequency (UHF) radiowaves as an adjunct is now being suggested.

This radiowave therapy targets all cancers, and irrefutable

proof on the success of hyperthermia treatment combined with radiation has been reported for the following nine tumour areas:

- Head and neck
- GBM
- Breast
- Rectum
- Melanoma
- Bladder
- Oesophagus
- Cervix
- Sarcomas

In advanced high-risk prostatic cancer, hyperthermia is feasible and well tolerated.[63]

Formerly of the United Kingdom and having practised in Western Australia, Dr John Holt has been conducting research and treatment for over thirty years. He became intrigued when his father, in his thirties at the time, was successfully treated for cancer of the eye in Paris by Dr Andre Denier, who used hyperthermia treatment. Holt's father had the eyeball removed in his teenage years but the cancer continued to grow. After Denier's therapy he lived into his eighties.

Holt was led to investigate further treatments in regard to electrical energy in the quest to cure cancer. Working with UHF, 434 MHz radiowaves, Holt is known for his additional use of a glucose-blocking agent now being researched in Ireland and India. Some clinics use treatment methods that utilise hyperthermia on its own and others combine it with low-dose radiation. The clinical studies clearly show that UHF radiowaves enhance the efficacy of radiation and chemotherapy.

Dr Jacobi van der Zee of the Daniel den Hoed Cancer Centre in Rotterdam, and other doctors in the United States and Japan, have worked together on clinical trials. Van der Zee demonstrated that the use of UHF, plus low-dose radiation, is a considerable improvement on conventional therapies without the often devastating side effects.[64] She has been working in this area for almost thirty years, with her research being backed by the Dutch government as well as the Dutch Cancer Council.

Beginning in early 2009, the Dutch government now reimburses citizens for hyperthermia therapy, the equivalent in Australia of a rebate (Medicare) from the federal government. This process, which has taken twenty years, acknowledges the work of Dr van der Zee and her colleagues.

Dr Sergio Maluta, head of the Radiation Oncology Department at the Azienda Ospedaliera Istituti Ospitalieri Di Verona, Italy is currently in discussions with the Italian government regarding rebates for the Italian people.

Currently the European Society for Hyperthermic Oncology (ESHO) is conducting a clinical trial across three countries on the best combination for the treatment of cancer using this fourth modality. The trials are being conducted in clinics in Verona in Italy; Munich, Berlin and Erlangen in Germany, and Rotterdam in the Netherlands. The twenty-fifth annual meeting of the ESHO is in Verona, Italy in June 2009.

Dr Nisar Syed, director of radiation oncology, and Dr Ajmel Puthawala of Long Beach Memorial Hospital in Los Angeles have nearly thirty years' experience using this therapy.

Jenny Barlow of Boggabri, Australia is working towards opening a clinic that uses hyperthermia combined with low-dose radiation, and at a later stage the glucose-blocking system. Barlow is also striving for government recognition to have this modality as a cancer treatment option available in Australia.[65]

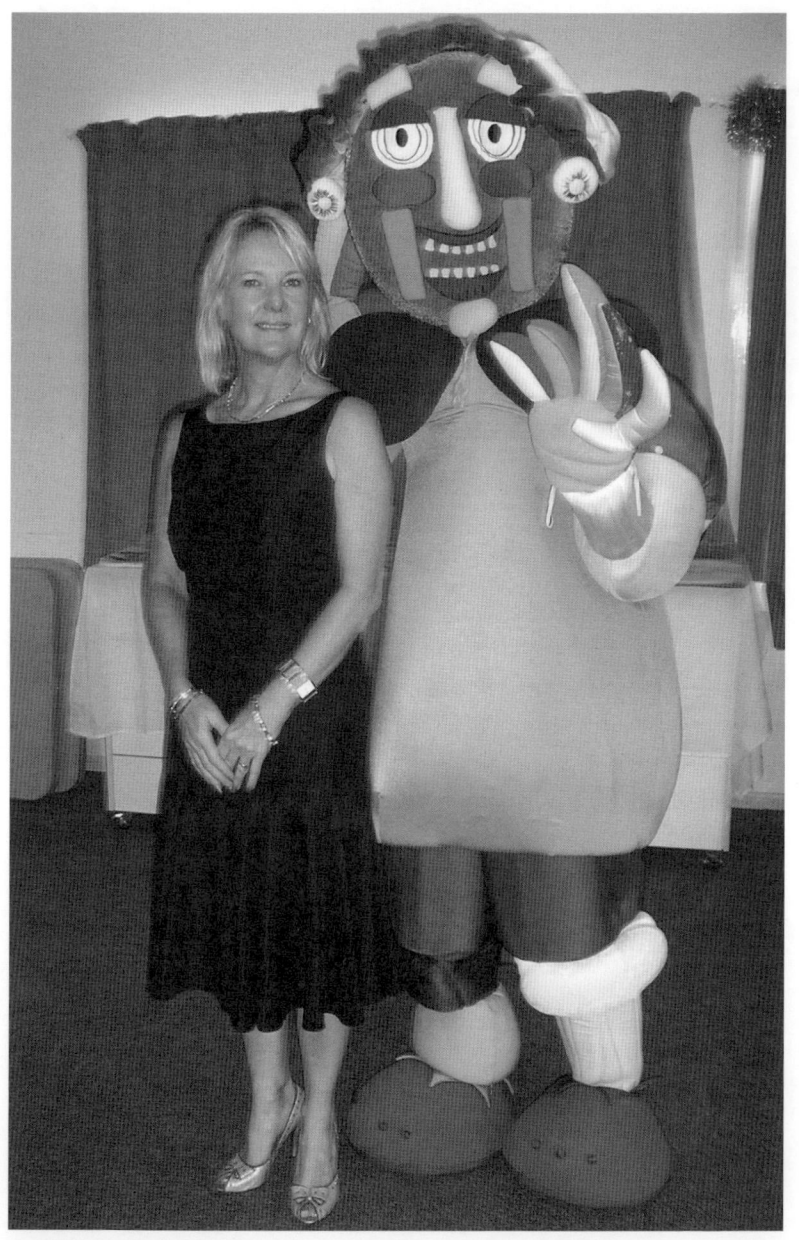

HEALTHY COMMUNITIES: As well as being aware of the benefits of eating healthy food, we must also be aware of electromagnetic fields and radiation.

CHAPTER 11

What You Can Do

Most employers and employees are unaware of how to deal with high incidences of cancer and cancers clusters in the workplace, as most people do not have an understanding of EMF/EMR. Also, the average person fails to understand the figures and technical language included in the reports. It is important to obtain advice from qualified private consultants who do not have a conflict of interest, and who specialise and are qualified in this area. Most electricians are also unaware of the relevant research.

Government standards in almost all countries are inappropriately high. For example, Australia's ELF EMF standard is currently 1000 mG units for the public and 5000 mG units for occupational settings. Investigative reports quote these standards,[66] which are the standards/guidelines for most countries, and the measurements do fall within federal guidelines. But it is important to understand that these figures do not relate to the biological effects. In other words, these fields can cause disease and cancer.

In practical terms, this means that you can be exposed to 999 mG units and the report will state that exposures are under the standard guidelines. You would not want to be exposed at this level for any length of time, however, and it is worth noting that high fields such as these occur quite often.

This has been happening for decades. I have witnessed

the investigative reports, and instances where employers and employees have been relieved that their exposure was below the standard. We cannot afford to remain uneducated on this topic. Fields of 2–4 mG units are deemed risky.

The Swedish Confederation of Professional Employees (TCO) has defined a worker-exposure standard of no more than 2mG units for EMF as the de facto standard. The Republic of Kazakhstan is the only country to have a standard for transient EMF: 50 GS units for industrial purposes. It is officially recognised in Kazakhstan that there is *no* safe level of exposure to transient EMF.

To help employers and employees gain some knowledge on the minimum testing[67] that would be required to assess an environment for dirty electricity, I include the following suggestions as guidance.[68] These procedures should also be carried out in the homes of all staff, particularly in their home offices and bedrooms:

- The STETZERiZER meter should be plugged into every power outlet in the building to give a reading of the transient EMF. In particular, the workstations of all employees should be measured. This is a simple process that gives an immediate reading. The figures on the meter will keep fluctuating. This procedure should be conducted several times a day for at least one working week. Ideally the reading should be no higher than 30 GS units. Filters must be installed to remove the dirty electricity transients.

    50 GS units is usually about 2 kHz and this harmful energy dissipates into the body at 1.7 kHz.

WHAT YOU CAN DO

- A gaussmeter should be used to measure the magnetic fields—ELF EMF—several times during the day, especially where all staff are located for long periods of time and also at chest level. A data logger should be left for a working week, to record where the employees spend most of their day. This should not be 'averaged' out over 24 hours or more.

The aim should be to work in fields no higher than 2 mG for extended periods of time. The BioInitiative Report recommends 1 mG for pregnant women and children.

FEMALE WORKERS

In laboratories, magnetic fields from 2 mG units–12 mG units have been found to block the action of melatonin, a hormone that is vital for protection against any cancer, and particularly breast cancer. High levels of melatonin are associated with a lower risk of breast cancer.

These magnetic fields have also been found to partially block the action of tamoxifen, a drug routinely used for the prevention and recurrence of breast cancer. Garland advised informing female employes about the tamoxifen research, and recommended that those who were taking the drug be transferred to a lower-current area if they so desired.

More detailed information about magnetic fields, breast cancer and melatonin is available in *Silent Fields: The Growing Cancer Cluster Story: When Electricity Kills.*

> **'Lee (2002) conducted a nested case-control study of residential and personal magnetic field exposures and spontaneous abortion. She reported that "women in the second through fourth quartiles of EMF exposure had a 50% increased risk of spontaneous abortion (RR = 1.5)".'**
>
> —David O Carpenter and Cindy Sage, 'Setting Prudent Public Health Policy for Electromagnetic Field Exposures' 2008[69]

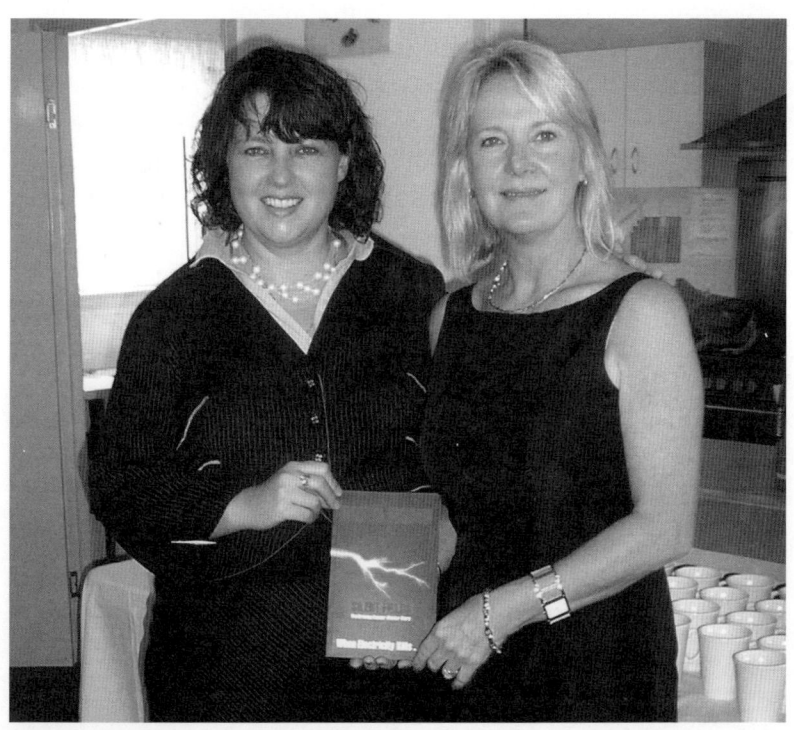

COMMUNITY HERO: The author with Annette Lourigan of Loganlea, Queensland, who is an expert at organising events.

CHAPTER 12

Cleaning Up Electricity

This issue is reminiscent of the battle to clean up the tobacco industry and manage the asbestos crisis, and will be no stranger to inaction by authorities and governments who, as tradition has shown, are slow to act on toxic agents. We have already gone too far down tobacco road. Asbestos was first discovered as a cause of illness in the early 1900s but was not recognised as an occupational hazard until 1936. It was not until 1995 that a conclusive ban was placed on its use, manufacture and import.

After the release of *Silent Fields* I was given further information that led me to the missing link explaining why dirty electricity has been instrumental in the dramatic rise of many disease processes and cancer, particularly breast cancer.

You may not have electrical equipment that generates dirty electricity in your own home, yet dirty electricity may enter from other buildings—homes, workplaces, hospitals and manufacturing plants—along the streets and areas that share transformers and the power grid that ultimately supplies your power needs. This dirty electricity finds it easier to flow into the home rather than return through the transformer and onto the substation via the grid.

There is special concern that our children are being exposed far too frequently to these harmful higher-frequency fields, as children often sit for hours in front of the various units of electronic equipment that proliferate in our homes today. Virtually all of us are exposed.

We are living our lives with this dangerous poison continually in our bodies. Whatever the state of the immune system, an environment polluted by artificial radiation makes it weaker which prevents our critical repair processes operating in an orderly fashion to prevent cancer. 'It is believed that these radio frequencies use the bone marrow as their main conducting circuit within the body. The bone marrow is part of the immune system where antibodies, white blood cells and other essential "germ fighters" are generated.'[70]

Every building, whether it is a school, hospital, workplace or home, should install the appropriate filters to clean up electrical environments and reduce exposure to the harmful effects of dirty electricity. Proper installation of these filters is required for maximum benefit.

It is critical that our schools be equipped with appropriate filters, especially those with very young children. We know there is hope when the Ontario Secondary School Teachers' Federation acknowledges dirty electricity on its website.

It is also critical for hospitals to install appropriate filters throughout the whole building. Shielded isolation transformers are currently installed so surgery procedure areas in hospitals are protected from these dirty electricity transients having a negative effect on many delicate operations, for example, heart and eye operations. Recovering patients—and workers—should also be in an electrically clean environment.

Some anecdotal evidence suggests that people who have cancer remission are more likely to have the cancer return if they go back to work or live in an electromagnetically dirty environment. It may well be that malignant tissue absorbs more electromagnetic radiation and actually thrives on it.

It is believed that cancer needs an acidic environment in which to thrive; in an alkaline environment cancer growth is retarded. When STETZERiZER filters have been installed, people's pH levels have been shown to change in two hours from an acid state to an alkaline state.

DRAMATIC EFFECTS OF FILTERS

When I was finally able to obtain the STETZERiZER microsurge meter, the readings in my new home were over 1999 GS units in most rooms. I then installed the appropriate number of filters to get the number down to under 30 GS units. I have since measured many homes with the meter and have found most have very high readings.

Ideally, electrical equipment today should be properly fitted with the appropriate built-in filter (capacitor) so the dangerous electromagnetic radiation that this equipment generates is not penetrating unsuspecting people. The cost by manufacturers to properly filter electrical equipment would be minimal. Manufacturers worldwide must install proper filtering systems in all things electrical so their products are not only 'green' but also electrically clean.

There is no doubt that the honeymoon stage of our love affair with all things electrical should be over. Each time we purchase unfiltered electrical appliances or energy-efficient equipment and lighting we are adding to the dirty electricity plague.

As water can become polluted when it travels through a contaminated environment, so too can electricity. In our buildings the clean water comes in and the dirty water is sent out via a different pathway. Our electricity supply is contaminated, if any of the power delivered these days could indeed be considered clean. Dirty electricity is a massive problem for the power industry, costing billions each year. The power industry calls this menace 'dirty power'. It is considered electrical pollution when it impacts equipment, and electrical poisoning when it impacts living creatures.

Filtering our electricity is an engineering solution to an engineering problem. Newer technologies must be created that not only consider the health of the planet but also do not compromise the health of the people. Dr Magda Havas reports that many homes with solar panels have very high dirty electricity: solar converts DC (direct current) to AC (alternating current) with power inverters that put an enormous amount of dirty electricity on the lines and power grid.

Broadcast and mobile phone masts each have their own switch-mode power supply or rectifier that converts AC to DC. Wind turbines usually change the AC to DC and the DC back to AC, a huge variable-speed frequency drive that causes enormous problems.

When the dirty electricity is put on the grid it can be measured. It can also be measured on the ground for several kilometres from the source. The dirty electricity and ground current can, however, be eliminated with proper design.

Interestingly, Helen Murphy, who suffers from EHS, lives with power poles approximately 1.5 metres from her front fence. Even though high measurements of magnetic fields have been a concern, Helen contacted me after reading *Silent Fields*, which brought attention to the STETZERiZER filters, and advised me that after the filters were installed in her home her symptoms improved dramatically. Helen's story can be found on page 21.

LEADING THE WAY

My path, which is so often challenging, is full of highs and lows but at the moment I am encouraged by the quick comprehension of people when I lecture. Private primary schools in Queensland's southeast have comprehended very quickly the need for filters to clean their school's electrical environment. I have measured for dirty electricity in one of these schools, and of the sixteen rooms—not even half—investigated, two rooms had readings of over 1999 GS units, with the oldest buildings also having readings of over 1400

GS units. Several workplaces have now requested filters, with many private citizens installing filters in their homes.

One of the most recently constructed lavish 'green' resorts in the north of Queensland, Australia is now considering installing filters so their guests will reap the benefits of an electrically clean environment.

Electrohypersensitivity (EHS) is a syndrome that is severely debilitating for increasing numbers of the population, and those affected respond more severely, with obvious symptoms. Even though I personally am not electrohypersensitive, this invisible and silent radiation that I do not feel is, as with everyone else, still affecting sensitive bodily processes.

DETRIMENTAL HEALTH EFFECTS

Dr William Rae, a former surgeon from Texas, determined that his allergic and neurological symptoms were caused by the electromagnetic fields in the operating room. Rae established the Environmental Health Center Dallas, where his patients were tested through exposure to a spectrum of electromagnetic fields. It was done in such a fashion that they were unaware of the testing, proving that EHS is a real clinical entity.

Chronic fatigue syndrome has been found to be widespread in the electronics industry, particularly in IT workers in Silicon Valley. It has also been noted in Japan, where chronic fatigue syndrome and depression are rampant, that younger people are often showing deterioration of mental faculties similar to that of the elderly. The young are withdrawing from society and shutting themselves off in their rooms.

'About 70% of the withdrawn Japanese children have chronic fatigue syndrome (CFS) with reduced blood flow to the brain,' says Professor Teruhisa Miike of Kumamoto University Medical School. His investigation of cerebral blood flow among children failing to attend school showed reduced blood flow in 75 percent of the cases. Miike states that their failure to attend school is not a 'psychological problem' but a serious illness accompanied by disorders in central nervous system function and immune function.

This chronic fatigue syndrome may be caused by electromagnetic waves, according to a study by Ryoichi Ogawa, a physician in Kobe, who suggests that 'reduced cerebral blood flow may possibly result from the influence of electromagnetic waves from IT equipment'. Dr Ogawa noted that about 80 percent of his CFS patients were frequent users on a daily basis of mobile phones, personal computers, TV games and other IT devices.

The symptoms of EHS, chronic fatigue syndrome, fibromyalgia, and Gulf War Syndrome are all virtually identical to those of radio-frequency sickness. Many of the symptoms of electrohypersensitivity closely resemble the symptoms of multiple sclerosis.

ELECTRICAL SENSITIVITY

After speaking with many who are electrohypersensitive, I now understand how exposure to these artificial electromagnetic fields is dramatically affecting the quality of many people's everyday lives. Stetzer has observed sufferers of multiple chemical sensitivity (MCS) are no longer afflicted after installing filters which is supported by earlier Russian research.

We are all sensitive to EMR, and every person is affected by electrical poisoning. Exposure that does not lead to immediate symptoms can still result in cumulative damage that can cause serious disease. Next time the health complaints of a person in your workplace are shrugged off, be careful that this warning signal is not ignored. Pay attention, as it is most probably the dirty electrical environment that is also silently and unknowingly harming everyone in the office.

Every time I lecture I hear many stories. Whether it is because people live or work close to radar systems, signalling systems for trains, antennae for broadcast systems or telecommunications systems, or have worked in offices with concentrated areas of electrical equipment, they so often tell of unrealised dreams of having children, living healthy lives or being cancer free. Many take their own lives as they see it as their only way to stop the relentless bombardment from EMFs.

The first European EHS White Zone Health Zone eco-village should be completed by mid 2009. Located in the southeast of France, this village will have emergency accommodation for those with EHS who need somewhere to recuperate and heal, and chalets for permanent living.

In May 2009 Netherlands National Radiation Day was held and the Honorable Stacy Ritter, mayor of Broward County, Florida, proclaimed May 2009 Electromagnetic Sensitivity (EMS) Awareness Month a move also officially stamped by M Jodi Rell, Governor of Connecticut. The mayor states that as a result of global electromagnetic pollution, people of all ages in Broward County and throughout the world have developed the illness known as electromagnetic sensitivity, a chronic and painful condition of hypersensitive reactions to electromagnetic radiation in the environment. There is no known cure.

The symptoms of EMS include: dermal changes; dermatitis; acute tingling and numbness; muscular weakness; headaches; heart rate changes; nausea; gastric problems; loss of visual acuity; severe neurological, respiratory and speech problems; and numerous other physiological symptoms. The Florida proclamation also states that EMS is 'a most devastating worldwide epidemic, the direct consequence of global exposures to electromagnetic radiation ...'[71]

The age of electricity, which has changed our lives dramatically, both industrially and personally, and allowed us to live virtual twenty-four-hour days has contributed significantly to death and serious disease. There has also been a parallel rise in leukaemia, brain tumours, breast cancer, diseases of the central nervous system, loss of fertility, prostate cancer, heart disease, miscarriage, depression and suicide. Altered sperm quality and quantity, and the subsequent effect on future generations are also areas of concern. Much of the increase in cardiovascular disease in the last fifty years is believed to be due to the adverse effects of electromagnetic radiation. In general, clinical exposure from EMF exposure resembles premature aging.[72]

ENCOURAGING SIGNS

In February 2009 a lawsuit was filed in District Court in Kansas City by the United States Justice Department on behalf of the Environmental Protection Agency. The EPA accused an energy company of failing to meet requirements of the Clean Air Act for more than a decade at a coal-fired power plant, stating that emissions from coal-fired power plants have detrimental effects on asthma sufferers, the elderly and children. These emissions have also been linked to air, water and ground pollution, according to the EPA.

The government estimates that coal-fired power plants account for nearly 70 percent of all sulphur dioxide emissions and 20 percent of nitrogen oxide emissions each year. It has become obvious we need to create cleaner power in our lives from the source to the end-point.

Until we put in place a technology that is green *and* clean I will continue to burn the midnight oil and listen to the cries of the people as they become increasingly aware, and as they become convinced that their ailments may be caused in part, or significantly influenced by, the dirty electricity plague. We filter our water to have cleaner water. There is no doubt that we must now filter our electricity for cleaner electricity. The installation of filters will also reduce our electricity bills.

The International Conference on Electromagnetic Fields and Human Health was held in Kazakhstan in September 2003.

In November of the same year the state health department of the Republic of Kazakhstan issued sanitary norms addressing the 1–400 kHz frequency.[73] A limit of 50 GS units (industrial) has since been mandated. As stated earlier, the republic has acknowledged that there is no safe level of exposure. For the public, a reading less than 30 GS units is more appropriate.

That Kazakhstan has already foreseen what a dramatic impact on the health of its citizens will be made by so quickly addressing the dirty electricity plague gives the hope that other countries will intelligently endorse the growing imperative to limit people's exposure.

As filters become more widely available globally in 2009,[74] a worldwide coalition with its roots in academia is currently being formed, acting on what one country has already endorsed as valid scientific fact. While filtering our electricity is not our only answer, its application is a huge step forward for civilisation.

As a major contributor to the cancer story, dirty electricity is the largest threat to our health that we have ever faced, as it is very much a part of our daily lives. It is in our homes, our workplaces, our schools and our hospitals. It is everywhere. This dirty electricity plague is bigger than all of us.

AFTERWORD

In 1956 Dr Alice Stewart discovered that a single exposure to a diagnostic X-ray shortly before birth will double the risk of an early cancer death, sparking controversy for decades. Today it is scientific fact that exposure to ionising radiation, even in low doses, can cause cancer. This is based on studies of Japanese bomb survivors, which showed that ionising radiation caused the dramatic increase in breast cancer and leukaemia, and on studies of in-utero irradiation of the foetus. Ionising radiation includes not only gamma rays from nuclear bombs but X-rays, CT scans and mammograms.

Apart from nuclear fallout, exposure to this form of radiation is by choice. The X-rays in the scanning equipment at Sydney Airport, Australia are being suggested as the cause of the current suspected breast cancer scare in airport employees.

Artificial radiation from non-ionising radiation also spells peril to our future children as well as to ourselves. Exposure to this form of radiation is on unsuspecting recipients. It is now widely acknowledged that non-ionising radiation can cause childhood leukaemia—the strongest evidence for a cancer is that the same cancer is significantly elevated in children. So is it any surprise that it can also cause breast cancer and other cancers?

Each one of us must become their own personal scientist and be willing to understand this artificial radiation that has been woven into our lives and viewed as a necessity by many. Exposure to non-ionising radiation includes:

- ELF EMF: power lines, substations, electrical wiring
- Transient EMF: transients on our electrical wiring (dirty electricity)
- RF EMF/MW: TV, radio and other broadcast antennae,

radar, mobile phones, mobile phone masts, wireless internet and other wireless devices

With magnetic resonance imaging (MRI) scans, the body is placed in a rapidly changing magnetic field and pulses of radio frequency are then applied. Microwaves are also used for communications. RF and MW emissions overlap considerably.

Whether the reading is for ELF EMF (measured in mG units) or transient EMF (measured in GS units), there is no safe exposure. Our personal choices are our own to make, yet it is vital that we all become educated to understand when we are being exposed and what we are willing to be exposed to. If one has a certain amount of exposure to one form of artificial radiation, it should be balanced by lessening exposures in other areas, that is, if we really wish to be irradiated at all.

ELF EMF and RF EMF have very similar biological effects in the body:[75]

- Genetic effects
- Cancer
- Cellular/molecular effects
- Electrophysiology
- Behaviour
- Nervous system
- Blood/brain barrier
- Calcium
- Cardiovascular
- Warm sensation
- Hormones
- Immunology
- Metabolic rate/effects
- Reproduction/growth
- Subjective symptoms
- Stress

Transient EMF generated in the intermediate frequency at the lower end of RF has characteristics of both ELF EMF and RF EMF. Transient EMF, with its own additional characteristics, is a parasite riding along our 50/60 Hz wiring and spiking up into RF EMF, exacerbating the adverse effects associated with ELF EMF and RF EMF. Milham commented that it is possible for some of the effects attributed to the magnetic fields from electricity to come from these transients. Transient EMF, together with the escalation of other cancers and diseases, would explain to a large extent the dramatic rise in breast cancer; in part the dramatic rise in diabetes; the sudden appearance of CFS; and more people experiencing EHS since dirty electricity was introduced in the 1970s.

Silent Fields was written due to my exasperation at the incomplete investigation of the electrical environment regarding the breast cancer cluster at the Toowong ABC TV studios in Australia.

I await with great curiosity the final investigative report on breast cancer cases—'significantly more than would have been expected by chance'[76]—across the other side of the globe at the University of California, San Diego that I discussed in chapter 1 of this book. While waiting for the final report, the elevators in the building at this university have meanwhile been shut down and several offices on the first floor have been vacated. All the power for the building passes though a small electrical room on the first floor, which is next to the elevator equipment room and the powerful motors that draw huge amounts of kilowatts. Both of those rooms are less than thirty metres away from where many of the women with breast cancer worked, according to Garland's report.

This breast cancer cluster is now being investigated by Leeka Kheifets, professor-in-residence, Department of Epidemiology, School of Public Health, who has a position at the University of California, Los Angeles. The report will be of interest as Slesin comments that Kheifets has spent most of her professional career either directly or indirectly working for Electric Power Research Institute, an arm of the electric utility industry.

Twenty-three years after the atomic bombs were dropped in 1945, it was confirmed and quantified in 1968 that ionising radiation (gamma rays) released from the bombs can cause breast cancer.[77] It was many years before Western scientists acknowledged that the resulting sickness came from the radiation from the bombs. It took many decades for scientists to understand how this affected our bodies.

The EMF (non-ionising radiation) breast cancer connection in women has been hotly debated since the first study reporting a connection in the Western world in 1982. The study was initially intended to look at the overall cancer risk in adults, but found accelerated development and growth of breast cancer, particularly among women younger than fifty-five years.[78] (An increase in excess cancers of the nervous system, uterus, and lymphoid tumours in adults was also indicated.) It is now twenty-seven years on and millions of lives have been lost to this devastating disease and other cancers. How many more have to die needlessly before dirty electricity is acknowledged as a contributing factor in breast cancer development?

When three cases of male breast cancer showed up in the same small office in Albuquerque in 2001, Dr Sam Milham testified for the men, arguing that the cancers were caused, in part at least, by EMFs from an electrical vault that was next to the basement office where the men worked. Milham commented in 2006 that after Gene Matanoski first announced an EMF–male breast cancer link in 1991, there have been fourteen additional studies reporting a similar association. Conducting further analysis in 1997, Dr Thomas Erren, Institute and Policlinic for Occupational and Social Medicine, University of Cologne, Germany determined that an ELF EMF–male breast cancer association is supported.[79] Due to the breast cancer risks attributed to reproductive factors, it is easier for the EMF association in women to be masked.

The rise of breast cancer incidence has accompanied the rise in our use of electricity. The introduction of dirty electricity and computers has accompanied the dramatic rise in breast cancer since the 1970s. Even though screening and better treatment methods are now engaged, breast cancer incidence is still rising.

Genetics and risk factors aside, like the ABC TV studios breast cancer cluster in Australia, there is a definite cause to the breast cluster in San Diego. There is already ample evidence in Garland's report that implicates a dirty electrical environment. Dirty electricity is contributing to breast cancer development and the development of other cancers. We now know that dirty electricity is most definitely penetrating the body at 1.7 kHz, which is why the Republic of Kazakhstan acted so quickly.

Already it is too late for millions of women and men. Millions of dollars are raised worldwide to find a cure for breast cancer yet we must also take simple steps in our daily lives to stop our breasts being irradiated. This may inconvenience us, and our employers, at times and may turn our lives upside down while we change ingrained habits and our working lives but we must not allow this to stop us from working through this dirty electricity plague together. There should be no doubt about the validity of Dr Robert Becker's belief that these silent fields are a competent cause for the origin of cancers.

> **If Alice Stewart had discovered that radiation was good for you, she might have won the Nobel Prize, as more than one of her admirers has commented. But since she is the bearer of bad news there's been a tendency to ignore her.**
>
> —Gayle Green, *The Woman Who Knew Too Much.*

APPENDIX A

Electromagnetic Frequencies

Extremely low frequency (ELF) 0–300 Hz
power lines, wiring in walls
Ultra-low frequency (ULF) 300 Hz–3 kHz
Very low frequency (VLF) 3–30 kHz
Low frequency (LF) 30–300 kHz
Medium frequency (MF) 300 kHz–3 MHz
AM radio
High frequency (HF) 3–30 MHz
AM radio, CB radio
Very high frequency (VHF) 30–300 MHz
FM radio, TV
Ultra-high frequency (UHF) 300–3000 MHz
mobile phones
Super-high frequency (SHF) 3–30 GHz
corresponds roughly to microwave band, satellite communication
Extremely high frequency (EHF) 30–300 GHz
Infrared radiation 300 GHz–810 THz
Visible light 810–1620 THz
Ultraviolet radiation 1620 THz–30 PHz
X-rays 30 PHz–30 EHz
Gamma rays 30–3000 EHz
nuclear bombs

APPENDIX B

Legal Advice to the Power Industry

WATSON & RENNER

Privileged Attorney-Client Communication

14 June 2002

FOR: UHSG Members

RE: EMF Science Reviews

We attach an updated list of EMF science reviews conducted by scientific panels, public health organizations, or governmental bodies. Since 1977, there have been 113 such reviews. The attached report lists these reviews, along with representative conclusions from each review. While each review includes many conclusions, the quotes from each review are representative of the overall conclusions(s) reached in that review.

We believe this list of science reviews and their key conclusions is useful information to consider in assessing the development of the EMF issue, and in preparing public disclosures and communications materials.

In the past, it was possible to preface the list with a statement that:

> "none of these reviews has concluded that exposure to power-frequency EMF causes cancer or any other disease."

We believe such a representation is no longer advisable because of the release of the California Department of Health (CDHS) "Fourth and Final Draft" report on EMF research (see #111 on attached list). The CDHS draft report concludes in part that:

> "To one degree or another all three of the DHS scientists are inclined to believe that EMFs <u>can cause</u> some degree of increased risk of childhood leukemia, adult brain cancer, Lou Gehrig's Disease, and miscarriage." (Emphasis added).

The final CDHS report is expected to contain the same statement.

> It is possible to argue that the CDHS conclusion does not say explicitly that there is an established cause and effect relationship between EMF and any disease. We believe, however that the CDHS conclusion is sufficiently close to causation that a global statement that none of the science reviews concludes there is a causal relationship would be legally inadvisable.

1919 M Street, NW, Washington, DC 20036 202 737 6302
CRENNER@W-R.COM Fax: 202 737 7611

APPENDIX C

For the Technically Minded

Dirty electricity is poor power quality and refers to an electrical signal that deviates from a normal 50/60 Hz sine wave. The technical term for dirty electricity—an unwanted modulation that is contaminating our electrical supply—is 'high-frequency voltage transients', as it rides along our electrical wiring. Dirty electricity can be picked up by the power lines delivering electricity to the home from the utility. Incorrect wiring, poor power quality, unbalanced electrical loads and interruptions to the flow of electrical current create continuous spikes (transients) up into this higher and more dangerous frequency, which is radio-frequency radiation. The electrical utility industry refers to these transients as 'dirty power'.

Dirty electricity—transient EMF—flows along wires and has characteristics of ELF EMF (extremely low frequency electromagnetic fields) and RF EMF (radio-frequency electromagnetic fields). Dirty electricity can even extend into radio frequencies above several MHz and can often get into the microwave range of the electromagnetic spectrum:

Transient EMF
ELF EMF   VLF   LF   RF EMF/MW

Virtually all of today's energy-efficient electronic devices are drawing their needs intermittently, inducing high levels of high-frequency harmonics and distortion back into a building's electrical system, thus creating dirty electricity. Devices are using more pulsed power and various forms of switching power supplies with transformers that convert our AC current to the low-voltage DC power used to power all our electronics. The appliances convert the AC they are receiving to DC, which the equipment will use to power its activities using less electricity. In this process, high frequencies are produced that go out onto the electrical circuit and cause high-frequency electromagnetic waves to radiate out from the circuits.

Some of the high frequencies produced are radiowave and microwave frequencies that disseminate their energy through the air rather than follow the electrical circuits. Dirty electricity is also the result of interrupted current generated by electrical appliances and equipment resulting in spikes. In the process of saving energy, these energy-efficient DC devices chop up the conventional AC 50/60 Hz sine waves and create electrical transients.

Transients are large, very brief increases in voltage: distortions in the sine wave that occur when electrical equipment is switched on and off, interrupting the electrical current flow. Transients have the effect of creating a high-frequency signal that is superimposed on the 50/60 Hz signal, creating 'parasitic oscillations' that ride on top of the existing 50/60 Hz power.

Technology is now in intermittent use, which means that it is switching on and off and adding to the spikes. Our electricity and power systems, which were originally generated at continuous use, have not kept up with the increasing demands being placed on them to handle modern appliances and equipment that operate at higher frequencies.

Examples of modern-day equipment designed to operate with interrupted current flow are: dimmer switches, which interrupt the current twice per cycle, or 120 times per second (it takes a lot of electrical energy to dim the light, and this 'excess light' is converted to radio frequencies); energy-efficient compact fluorescent lighting (20,000 times per second); halogen lamps; and all equipment produced since the 1980s that uses switching power supplies.

The more that electricity deviates from the 50/60 Hz sine wave the poorer the power quality and the more dirty the electricity. High-frequency dirty electricity generated by electrical equipment in buildings travels along the electrical distribution system in and between buildings and through the ground. Dirty electricity generated outside the building enters the building on electrical wiring, and through ground rods and conductive plumbing. Humans and conducting objects in contact with the ground become part of the circuit.

The STETZERiZER filter contains an electrical capacitor that shorts out the harmful high-frequency transients and harmonics on the circuit that contributes to poor power quality.

Surges in power came along with computer use, with surge protectors created to prevent computers from crashing. Computers generate at higher frequencies and the power surges occurred due to our 50/60 Hz wiring being polluted by these higher frequencies. What is now known is that this energy from the computer is coupled to our bodies by the capacitance—a measure of the capacitor's ability to store charge—between our bodies and the electrical wires within the walls of our buildings. The body works on DC current but the currents from our wiring introduce AC currents into our systems, interrupting our natural bodily signals.

These higher frequencies are more likely to penetrate living organisms as they have more energy than ELF EMF in the 50/60 Hz range. Energy is proportional to frequency: the energy is 1,000 times higher at 60 kHz than it is at 60 Hz. These surges of radio-frequency energy can contain up to 2,500 times the energy of 50/60 Hz.

Russia and other Eastern bloc countries allow 25 volts per metre of exposure up to, but not including, 2 kHz in an electrical field. At 2 kHz and above, they allow only 2.5 volts per metre. There is not ten times more energy between 1.9 kHz and 2.1 kHz, yet the standard for exposure is dropped by a factor of ten. The reason is that the energy is now being dissipated inside the human body.

Dirty electricity helps to explain the inconsistencies between the real-world studies versus the laboratory studies, where a pure 50/60 Hz sine wave is used.

APPENDIX D

How Clean is Our Lighting?[80]

In 1879 Thomas Edison successfully developed the electric light bulb and we have since witnessed many changes to our lighting systems. Research is currently being conducted to further our understanding of how inappropriate and inappropriately timed lighting plays a role in the cancer story; whether there is a correlation between countries with the highest level of exposure to artificial light at night and rising cancer statistics.

The increase in melanoma since the 1950s cannot be adequately explained by environmental exposure to ultraviolet radiation. The increased rate of melanoma predates the decline in ozone (the depletion of the ozone layer results in increased levels of UV reaching the earth) and we must have further understanding of the effects of decreased exposure to natural sunlight and over-exposure to artificial lighting. The hazards attributed to electricity and its by-products—artificial electromagnetic fields and artificial lighting—will eventually be acknowledged as part of the cancer story.

In the rush to be seen as green, governments are embracing any technology that promises to reduce consumption of fossil fuels and emission of greenhouse gases. The move to compact fluorescent lighting (CFL) indicates the failure to understand that this form of lighting is a huge contributor to dirty electricity. This form of lighting is very dangerous to our health: a typical electronically ballasted CFL operates in the 24–100 kHz frequency range: the dirty electricity range.

Some epileptics are also reporting effects from this new form of lighting and blood glucose levels have been shown to rise in diabetics solely from sitting near a lamp with a CFL for a few hours.

CLED (clean LED) lighting is now available to replace CFLs and incandescent bulbs. A light bulb used for alleviating arthritis (8–10 minutes daily) is also available in this range.

CLED LIGHTS (CLEAN LED LIGHTS) AC DIRECT-VOLTAGE INPUT LED TUBE LIGHTS

Health considerations

- These generally have the lowest magnetic fields of all forms of electronic parts, including bulbs for lighting, and they match incandescent bulb emissions.
- They emit no UV or IR wavelengths but can be tailored to emit a single wavelength or full visible-light spectrum wavelengths.
- They do not generate dirty power.

Environmental Considerations

- They require no ballast, transformers or controllers for operation as electronic parts do emit harmful EM/RF fields. CLEDs have no transformer converting from AC to DC.
- They last fifty times as long as incandescent light bulbs, saving resources and energy in manufacture.
- LEDs are 90+ percent more energy efficient than incandescent light bulbs and produce fewer greenhouse gases.
- Their initial cost is higher than other lighting but LEDs are more cost effective over the lifetime of the lights.
- They contain no harmful materials and are completely biodegradable and recyclable.
- They do not generate dirty power.

Governments should insist that manufacturers produce light bulbs that do not contain toxic chemicals and are electromagnetically clean (do not produce RF or UV radiation); in other words, light bulbs that are safe for the environment and for human health.

INCANDESCENT LIGHTS

The original incandescent light bulbs generate heat in the form of infrared radiation that makes them energy inefficient.

Health Considerations
- These lights generally have the lowest magnetic fields of all forms of lighting.

Environmental Considerations
- They do not contain any harmful chemicals.
- They use more energy than CFLs and generally don't last as long.
- They can be disposed of in landfill or recycled.

FLUORESCENT LIGHTS

These lights emit much higher magnetic fields than incandescent light bulbs at around 20–100 mG units.

Health Considerations
- They contain toxic PCBs.
- They emit UV radiation.
- They have been associated with malignant melanomas.
- People with sensitivities to EMR report discomfort or intolerance to this form of lighting.
- Flickering fluorescent lights have triggered epilepsy.
- Fluorescent lighting has been associated with hyperactivity, irritability, fatigue and attention disorders.

Environmental Considerations
- They contain around 30 mg of mercury.
- There are disposal concerns for landfill.

HALOGEN LIGHTS

These lights generally emit higher magnetic fields than incandescent light bulbs because they contain transformers.

Health Considerations
- They emit UV radiation.

Environmental Considerations
- One of the most energy-consuming forms of lighting available.

COMPACT FLUORESCENT LIGHTS (CFLs)

These lights generally emit higher magnetic fields than incandescent light bulbs.

Health Considerations
- People with sensitivities to EMR report discomfort or intolerance to this form of lighting.
- They produce dirty electricity on wires and radio frequencies through air; they generate radio frequency radiation (RF). They also generate UV radiation. The frequencies of RF and UV have been associated with adverse health in numerous peer-reviewed scientific studies, and a growing number of people are reporting that these bulbs make them ill.

Environmental Considerations
- These lights contain an average of 5 mg of mercury.
- CFLs are 80 percent more energy efficient than

incandescent light bulbs and produce fewer greenhouse gases.
- They last fifteen times as long as incandescent globes, saving resources and energy in manufacture.
- There are disposal concerns for landfill.

Not all energy-efficient light bulbs are the same. Some do not contribute to dirty electricity or produce radio frequencies. Test the bulb for radiation with a portable radio. If the radio buzzes, do not use the bulb.

FULL-SPECTRUM FLUORESCENT LIGHTS

These lights mimic natural sunlight in that they contain the full spectrum of sunlight's frequencies and are therefore claimed to be both natural and beneficial for health.

Health considerations
- Studies have shown improvements to health and behaviour.
- Some produce high frequencies that affect those with EHS.

Environmental considerations
- These lights contain mercury.
- There are disposal concerns for landfill.

NOTE: Mercury is the most toxic heavy metal and one of the most toxic substances known—it is even more toxic than arsenic. It is contained in CFLs and all other types of fluorescent lights and is emitted by power stations in the process of generating electricity. One gram of mercury contaminates one billion litres of water.[81]

APPENDIX E

Signees to the Venice Resolution[82]

Pasquale Avino, Italian National Institute for Prevention and Worker Safety, Rome, Italy

Alessandro d'Alessandro, ICEMS, MD, Benevento, Italy

Angelico Bedini, Italian National Institute for Prevention and Worker Safety, Rome, Italy

Igor Belyaev, associate professor in toxicological genetics, Department of Genetics, Microbiology and Toxicology, Stockholm University, Stockholm, Sweden

Fiorella Belpoggi, ICEMS, vice scientific director, European Foundation for Oncology and Environmental Sciences 'B Ramazzini', Bologna, Italy

Carl Blackman, ICEMS; president, Bioelectromagnetics Society (1990–91), Raleigh, North Carolina, USA

Martin Blank, Department of Physiology and Cellular Biophysics, Columbia University, New York, USA

Natalia Bobkova, ICEMS, Institute of Cell Biophysics, Pushchino, Moscow Region

Bill Bruno, Theoretical biophysics, earned at Department of Physics, University of California, Berkeley, USA

Zhaojin Cao, National Institute Environmental Health, Chinese Center for Disease Control, China

Simona Carrubba, PhD, Louisiana State University Health Sciences Center, Shreveport, Louisiana, USA

Catarina Cinti, ICEMS, director, National Research Center, Institute of Clinical Physiology, Siena, Italy

Mauro Cristaldi, DipBAU, Universita degli Studi 'La Sapienza', Roma, Italia

Suleyman Dasdag, Biophysics Department of Medical School, Dicle University, Diyarbakir, Turkey

Antonella De Ninno, ICEMS, Italian National Agency, Energy, Environment and Technology, Frascati, Italy

Emilio Del Giudice, ICEMS, International Institute of Biophysics, Neuss, Germany

Alvaro de Salles, ICEMS, Universidade Federal do Rio Grande do Sul, Porto Alegre, Brazil

Sandy Doull, Consultant, Noel Arnold and Associates, Box Hill, Victoria, Australia

Christos Georgiou, ICEMS, professor of biochemistry, Department of Biology, University of Patras, Greece

Reba Goodman, professor emeritus, Clinical Pathology, Columbia University, New York, USA

Settimo Grimaldi, ICEMS, Institute of Neurobiology and Molecular Medicine, National Research, Rome, Italy

Livio Giuliani, ICEMS spokesman; deputy director, National Institute of Prevention and Worker Safety, East Veneto and South Tirol, Camerino University, Italy

Lennart Hardell, ICEMS, Department of Oncology, University Hospital, Orebro, Sweden

Magda Havas, ICEMS, Environmental and Resource Studies, Trent University, Ontario, Canada

Gerard Hyland, ICEMS, International Institute of Biophysics, Neuss, Germany

Antonella Lisi, ICEMS Institute of Neurobiology and Molecular Medicine, National Research Council, Rome, Italy

Louisanna Ieradi, Istituto per lo Studio degli Ecosistemi CNR, Roma, Italia

Olle Johansson, assoc prof, Experimental Dermatology Unit, Department of Neuroscience, Karolinska Institute, Stockholm

Vini G Khurana, neurosurgeon, Canberra Hospital and associate professor of neurosurgery, Australian National University Medical School

Henry Lai, ICEMS, Department of Bioengineering, University of Washington, Seattle, USA

Lukas Margaritas, professor of cell biology and radiobiology, Athens University, Athens, Greece

Fiorenzo Marinelli, ICEMS, Institute of Molecular Genetics National Research Council, Bologna Italy

Andrew A Marino, professor, Department of Orthopaedic Surgery, Louisiana State University, Shreveport, Louisiana, USA

Vera Markovic, Faculty of Electrical Engineering, University of Nis, Serbia

Ed Maxey, MD, retired surgeon, Fayetteville, Arkansas, USA

Gerd Oberfeld, Public Health Department, Salzburg State Government, Salzburg, Austria, speaker for environmental medicine, Austrian Medical Association, Vienna, Austria

Jerry Phillips, director, Science Learning Center, University of Colorado, Colorado Springs, Colorado, USA

Elihu Richter, ICEMS, head, Occupational and Environmental Medicine, Hebrew University-Hadassah, Israel

Leif Salford, ICEMS, professor and chairman, Department of Neurosurgery, Lund University, Sweden

Massimo Scalia, professor of evolution models in applied sciences, Mathematical Physical and Natural Science, University of 'La Sapienza', Rome, Italy

Nesrin Seyhan, ICEMS, head, Department of Biophysics; director, Gazi NIRP Center, Ankara, Turkey

Zamir Shalita, consultant on electromagnetic hazards, Ramat Gan, Israel

Morando Soffritti, ICEMS, scientific director, European Foundation for Oncology and Environmental Sciences, 'B Ramazzini', Bologna, Italy

Stanley Szmigielski, ICEMS, Military Institute of Hygiene and

Epidemiology, Warsaw, Poland
Ion Udroiu, Italian National Institute for Prevention and Worker Safety, Rome, Italy
Clarbruno Verduccio, Prof Lt Col Commander CF, Marine Military, La Spezia, Italy
Mehmet Zeyrek, professor of physics, Middle East Technical University, Ankara, Turkey
Mikhail Zhadin, ICEMS, honorary scientist of Russian Federation, Institute of Cell Biophysics, Pushchino, Russia
Stylianos Zinelis, MD, ICEMS, vice president, Hellenic Cancer Society, Cefalonia, Greece
Anna Zucchero, ICEMS, MD, Internal Medicine Department, Venice-Mestre Hospital, Venice, Italy

Additional signees who are qualified but have not published EMF papers, or have not published prior to 2000:

Stéphane Egot-Lemaire, post-doctoral researcher, Institute for Science and Technology in Medicine, Keele University Medical School, Staffordshire, UK
Andrew Goldsworthy, lecturer in biology (retired), Imperial College London, UK
Sarah J Starkey, PhD, neuroscience, University of London, London, UK

RESOURCES

SURETOUCH VISUAL MAPPING SYSTEM

For updated information on the growing number of clinics using this technology worldwide, go to: www.suretouch.com.au

Australia

At the time of publication, Dr Graeme Langsford, the first in Australia to operate this system, has been performing these tests for more than a year.

Breast Centre Benowa
122 Ashmore Road
Benowa
Queensland

Phone +61 7 5539 3999

New Zealand

Burton King is a breast and general surgeon, and fellow of the Royal Australasian College of Surgeons.

Glenmore Surgeons
153 Glenmore Street
Kelburn
Wellington 6012

Phone +64 4 475 7670 or +64 4 475 7674

United States

Medical Tactile Inc
Suite 600
5757 Century Blvd
Los Angeles
California 90045

Phone +1 310 641 8228

THE STETZERiZER METER AND FILTERS

The STETZERiZER meter is the only meter of its type in the world. This proven STETZERiZER system is simple to operate so anyone can clean their electrical environment in any building, whether it is at their home, workplace, school, university or hospital. As the filters become more easily available worldwide a list of points of purchase is being compiled. Contact the author at: donnafisher@silentfields.com for further information.

CLED LIGHTING

CLEDs are recommended in 'Public Health SOS: The Shadow Side of the Wireless Revolution: 110 Questions on Electromagnetic Pollution', from a forum at the Commonwealth Club of California. As these become more easily available worldwide, a list of distributors is being compiled.

To find out points of purchase please contact the author at: donnafisher@silentfields.com

GLOSSARY

cancer cluster A greater than expected number of cases of a particular disease in a group of people in a geographical area, or over a period of time.

capacitive coupling Use of a capacitor to transfer energy from one circuit to another.

DECTs Digitally enhanced cordless phones.

dirty power Term used by the power industry. The alternate term used by the scientists is dirty electricity.

electrohypersensitivity (EHS) A condition where individuals experience adverse health effects while using or being in the vicinity of devices emanating electric, magnetic or electromagnetic fields (EMFs). Whatever its cause, EHS is a real and sometimes debilitating problem for the affected persons, while the level of EMF in their neighbourhood is no greater than is encountered in normal living environments.

electromagnetic spectrum A group of distinct energy forms that emanate from various sources: the energies released are referred to as types of EMR.

ELF Extremely low frequency (often termed extra-low frequency). The newer term, weak low intensity EMF, is also being used.

ELF EMF Covers the frequency range of 3–300Hz.

EMF Electric, magnetic and electromagnetic fields associated with electricity, whether it is from artificially created (man-made) sources such as power generation or from natural processes going on within animal or plant cells.

EME Electromagnetic energy (often used for EMF/EMR).

epidemiology A study of the various factors influencing the occurrence, distribution, prevention and control of disease, injury, and other health-related events in a defined human population. Epidemiological studies imply the analysis of a statistical connection between exposure and disease. A statistical connection does not mean that the exposure causes the disease.

frequency The number of complete cycles of an electromagnetic wave in a second. Unit: hertz. Abbreviation: Hz. 1 Hz = 1 cycle per second.

genotoxic Any evidence of genetic damage, cell death or neoplastic transformation. Any substance that damages DNA or chromosomes. A genotoxic substance is mutagenic, carcinogenic and teratogenic. Genotoxic substances can cause cancer, reproductive health effects and neurological damage.

glioma tumour Glioblastoma is a very aggressive and fatal brain tumour.

harmonic Multiples of the original frequency.

ionising radiation Electromagnetic radiation with photon energy high enough to break molecular bonds and damage genetic material. Gamma rays and X-rays are examples.

milliGauss; mGauss; mG Measurement of a magnetic field. A milliGauss is a measure of ELF intensity, and is used to describe electromagnetic fields from appliances, power lines, interior electrical wiring, etc.

MW; microwave Technology that operates at this frequency includes mobile phones, microwaves, telecommunications links, radar, satellite communications, weather-observation equipment and medical diathermy. Because microwaves are also used for communication, RF and MW emissions overlap considerably. Microwave energy is within the radio frequency band of the electromagnetic spectrum and ranges from 300 MHz–300 GHz.

non-ionising radiation The part of the electromagnetic spectrum extending from zero frequency to the frequencies of visible light.

precautionary principle The principle states that when there are indications of possible adverse effects, though they remain uncertain, the risks from doing nothing may be far greater than the risks of taking action to control these exposures. The precautionary principle shifts the burden of proof from those suspecting a risk to those who discount it.

rad; radiation absorbed dose A measurement that calculates the amount of radiation absorbed by body tissues.

radar Radar system has a transmitter that emits either microwaves or radiowaves that are reflected by the target and detected by a receiver.

radiation The energy transmitted by waves that travels and spreads out as it goes.

resonance The tuning of a biological response to an external signal. Resonance can also be applicable to organs, tissues or other body parts.

radiofrequency radiation; RFR Higher-frequency radiation used by communications systems. Used in technologies such as mobile communications, radios, TVs, paging antennae, computers. Radiofrequency radiation (RF) power density is measured in: volts per meter = 0.614 V/m or in microwatts per centimetre squared = 0.1 μW/cm2. In the United States and Canada, for example, the amount of allowable RF near a cell tower is one thousand microwatts per centimetre squared (1000 μW/cm2) for some mobile phone frequencies.

BIBLIOGRAPHY

Publications

Becker, R O, Dr. *Cross Currents: A Startling Look at the Effects of Electromagnetic Radiation on Your Health: The Perils of Electropollution, the Promise of Electromedicine*. Tarcher Putnam: USA 2000.

Davies, J. 'There are risks as well as benefits—so get the facts, then decide'. *The Scotsman*. Scotland 2009. See www.news.scotsman.com

Epstein, S D Dr, Bertell, R & Seaman, B. 'Dangers and unreliability of mammography: Breast examination is a safe, effective, and practical alternative'. *International Journal of Health Services*, 31(3): 605–615, 2001.

Evans, N. 'State of the evidence: What is the connection between the environment and breast cancer?' The Breast Cancer Fund USA 2004.

Genuis S J. 'Fielding a current idea: Exploring the public health impact of electromagnetic radiation.' *Public Health* (2007), doi: 10.1016/j.puhe. 2007.04.008.

Gray, J, PhD (ed). State of the Evidence: The Connection Between Breast Cancer and the Environment. The Breast Cancer Fund, USA 2008.

Havas, (assoc prof). 'Dirty electricity: An invisible pollutant in schools.' Environmental Resource Studies. Trent University, Ontario, Canada 2006. Sourced from http://biotech.about.com/gi/dynamic/offsite.htm?zi=1/xj&sdn=biotech&cdn=money&tm=8388&gps=219_27_1020_545&f=1

Havas, (assoc prof). Electrical Pollution Taskforce. Markham, Environmental Resource Studies. Trent University, Ontario, Canada 2005. Sourced from www.stop-emf.ca/stopinfo/HavasPresentationTaskForce.pdf

Havas, M (assoc prof). 'Power quality affects teacher wellbeing and student behavior in three Minnesota Schools'. *ScienceDirect*, Elsevier 2008. See www.dirtyelectricity.ca/images/08_HavasOlstad_schools1.pdf

Henshaw, D L (prof). 'What about the effect of EMFs on melatonin and breast cancer? A set of frequently asked questions specifically about melatonin.' Bristol University, UK 2006.

Johansson, O (assoc prof). 'The Effects of Radiation in the Cause of Cancer.' *Icon*, issue 4, 2005. See http://www.canceractive.com/page.php?n=967

Labi, Sharon. 'Unlocking the riddles of a condition that prefers to keep secrets.' Article published in the online journal *Nature* and reported in *The Sunday Telegraph*, 3 May 2009.

McLean, L. 'EMR and health: How green is your lighting?' *EMR and Health*, vol 3, no 3. Australia 2007.

Maret, K (MD). 'Electromagnetic fields and human health'. International conference Electromagnetic Fields and Human Health. Kazakhstan, September 2003.

Medical Tactile Imaging. SureTouch Visual Mapping System. 'Digital breast exam breakthrough: New technology for the early detection of breast cancer.' USA 2002.

Morgan, G, Ward, R and Barton, M. 'The contribution of cytotoxic chemotherapy to survival in adult malignancies.' Department of Radiation Oncology, Northern Sydney Cancer Centre, Royal North Shore Hospital, NSW, Australia 2004.

Rees C & Havas M. *Public Health SOS: The Shadow Side of the Wireless Revolution: 110 Questions on Electromagnetic Pollution*'. Commonwealth Club of California forum. Wide Angle Health, LLC. USA 2008.

Slesin, L. 'Faulty DNA repair may explain EMF role in childhood leukemia'. *Microwavenews*, vol XXVIII, no 10, December 2008. See www.microwavenews.com

Stevens, R G, Wilson B W and Anderson L E (eds). *The Melatonin*

Hypothesis: Breast Cancer and the Use of Electric Power. Columbus Battelle Press, USA 1997.

The National Foundation for Alternative Medicine USA. 'The health effects of electrical pollution.' The National Foundation for Alternative Medicine, USA.

Valentina, N. 'Occupational and population health risks of radio frequency electromagnetic fields'. Electromagnetic Fields and Human Health report, Kazakhstan 2003.

Zharkinov, E. 'Sickness rate of workers in electrolysis sections of titanic-magnesium and zinc industries of Kazakhstan report'. Electromagnetic Fields and Human Health conference, Kazakhstan 2003.

Websites

www.abc.net.au/news/stories/2008/11/25/2429401.htm?section=justin

www.buergerwelle.de/pdf/la_quinta_cancer_cluster.pdf

www.dirtyelectricity.ca/images/08_HavasOlstad_schools1.pdf

www.ecopolitan.com/health-resources/emfprotection/147-health-effects-radio

www.emfacts.com

www.electricalpollution.com.documents/08_Havas_UFL_SCENIHR.pdf

www.electricpollution.com/Lloyd_Morganexcerpts.htm

www.emfsolutions.ca/compact_fluorescent_bulbs_are_dangerous.htm

www.emrpolicy.org/public_policy/schools/magda_havas_hsn_presentation.pdf

http://www.europarl.europa.eu/sides/getDoc.do?pubRef=-//EP//TEXT+TA+P6-TA-2009-0216+0+DOC+XML+V0//EN

www.jerseymastconcern.co.uk

www.next-up.org

www.stop-emf.ca/stopinfo/HavasPresentationTaskForce.pdf
http://ww5.komen.org/ExternalNewsArchive.aspx
www.icems.eu
www.stop-emf.ca/stopinfo/HavasPresentationTaskForce.pdf

NOTES

Chapter 1

1 Genuis S J Fielding, 'A current idea: Exploring the public health impact of electromagnetic radiation.' Public Health (2007) oi:10.1016/j.puhe.2007, 04.008.
2 Electricity produces an electric and a magnetic field, which together are known as an electromagnetic field; milliGauss (mG) is the scientific term for the measurement of a magnetic field.
3 Lai and Singh, O'Neill, Svedenstal, Rudiger, Schar.
4 The full advice law firm from Watson and Renner, Washington DC to the electrical utilities worldwide is available in Appendix B. This private and confidential advice was obtained in a legal manner.
5 Becker, 1990, p 215.
6 A handful of other cancers, including ovarian and salivary gland cancers, have also been reported www.microwavenews.com

Chapter 2

7 Armstrong B et al, 1994. 'Association between exposure to pulsed electromagnetic fields and cancer in electric utility workers in Quebec, Canada and France.' *American Journal of Epidemiology*. 140, (9): 805-820).
8 Milham, S MD MPH and Morgan LL BS, 2008. 'A new electromagnetic exposure metric: High frequency voltage transients associated with increased incidence in teachers in a California school.' AM J Med, May 29:51 (8) 579-586.
9 Author's discussions with Dr Milham.

Chapter 3

10 For more in-depth information on Dr Havas' research and studies in schools see www.dirtyelectricity.ca/images/08_HavasOlstad_schools1.pdf

11   Havas, 2006, p 2.

Chapter 4
12   Gunter (PhD), H Strickler (MD) and colleagues at the Albert Einstein College of Medicine, New York.
13   Dr Magda Havas, Olstad 2008, p 2.

Chapter 5
14   Henshaw, 2006, p 6.
15   Gray, 2008, p 6.
16   At the September 2003 international conference which preceded Kazakhstan's move to issue sanitary norms (November 2003) to protect their citizens.
17   Maret, p 5, 2003.
18   Beniashvili et al. 2005. 'The effects of radiation in the cause of cancer', article specially written for ICON by Olle Johansson, associate professor of the Department of Neuroscience at the world famous Karolinska Institute. http://www.canceractive.com/page.php?n=967
19   Author of *Preventing Breast Cancer: The Story of a Major, Proven, Preventable Cause of this Disease.*
20   *The Times*, 19 February 2009.
21   SureTouch (2004) is currently approved by the Therapeutic Goods Administration in Australia as 'palpation imaging for the clinical breast exam'. SureTouch has been cleared for documenting palpable breast lesions by the United States Food and Drug Administration. The system has also gained European approval with the granting of its CE Mark. It is registered with the Ministry of Health in New Zealand and has recently been granted approval as a screening device by the State Food and Drug Administration in China.
22   *American Journal of Surgery*, 192 (2006) pp 444–449.
23   Evans, N. 2004, p 4.
24   The BioInitiative Report, a scientific review of over 2000 studies, 2007.

NOTES

Chapter 6

25 Firstenberg, A. 2006, p 5. 'The largest biological experiment ever', *Sun Monthly*, 1 Jan 2006.
26 'Cancer trends during the 20th century.' Örjan Hallberg MSc and associate professor Olle Johansson, 2002.
27 Firstenberg, A. 2006 p 5.
28 'Why people are worried about EMF: A UK perspective.' Eileen O'Connor of the UK Radiation Research Trust. Workshop on EMF and Health: Science and Policy, European Commission, Brussels, 11–12 February 2009.
29 Judgement of the Crown Court of Nanterre, France. 4 February 2009.
30 Judgement of The Tribunal de Grande Instance (District Court) of Carpentras, France, 16 February 2009.
31 http://www.europarl.europa.eu/sides/getDoc.do?pubRef=-//EP//TEXT+TA+P6-TA-2009-16+0+DOC+XML+V0//EN and http://www.europarl.europa.eu/sides/getDoc.do?pubRef=-//EP//TEXT+TA+P6-TA-2009-0216+0+DOC+XML+V0//EN
32 The e-book *Public Health SOS: The Shadow Side of the Wireless Revolution*, November 2008.
33 The blood/brain barrier is the same in a rat as it is in a human being.
34 Adapted from 'Children and mobile phones: The health of the following generations is in danger'. Russian National Committee on Non-Ionising Radiation Protection, Moscow, Russia, 14 April 2008.
35 Excerpt from transcript of Dr Carlo's meeting with Scrutiny Panel, www.jerseymastconcern.co.uk

Chapter 7

36 www.next-up.org

Chapter 8

37 Becker, 1990, p 257.

38 Becker, 1990, p 260.
39 *Journal of the Australasian College of Nutritional and Environmental Medicine*, November 2007, Vol 26, No 2, pages 3–7.
40 'New report on autism.' 20 November 2007. www.emfacts.com
41 Maret, K. p 9, 2003. 'Sickness rate of workers in electrolysis sections of titanic-magnesium and zinc industries of the Republic of Kazakhstan.'
42 Excerpts from transcript: Dr George Carlo's meeting with Scrutiny Panel. www.jerseymastconcern.co.uk
43 From an article published in the *American Journal of Epidemiology*, November 2008.
44 TNO Physics and Electronics Laboratory, The Netherlands, 2003. 'Effects of global communication system radio-frequency fields on wellbeing and cognitive functions of human beings with and without subjective complaints.' Netherlands Organization for Applied Scientific Research 1–63.
45 #821: Autism and DECT Baby Monitors, November 23 2007, www.emfacts.com
46 Rees C and Havas M. 2008, p 22.
47 Dr Magda Havas, *SOS: Public Health*, p 65.

Chapter 9

48 Lichtenstein P, Holm NV, Verkasalo PK, Iliadou A, Kaprio J, Koskenvuo M, et al. 'Environmental and heritable factors in the causation of cancer: Analyses of cohorts of twins from Sweden, Denmark and Finland.' N Engl J Med 2000:343:78–85.
49 Van-Steensil Moll et al 1985, Infante-Rivard, 1995.
50 Nordstrom and Nordensen et al 1983, 1984, 1988.
51 Spitz et al, Wilkins et al 1988.
52 Shen et al *Leukemia & Lymphoma* 2008.
53 This polymorphism/snp is known by a variety of

designations: 'Ex9+16G>A' and 'Arg280His'.
54 Juan Manuel Mejia-Arangure.
55 Slesin, 2008, p 1, microwavenews.com
56 Hallberg and Johansson report that deaths due to asbestosis were not known until after the 1960s despite the fact that asbestos has been used as a building material since the end of the 19th century.
57 *Journal of the Australasian College of Nutritional and Environmental Medicine*, Vol 21 No 2 April 2002.
58 Firstenberg, A, p 5, 2006.
59 Hallberg and Johansson, 2002b, 2004, 2005a.
60 Excerpted from 'The heath effects of electrical pollution', The National Foundation for Alternative Medicine, US. Originally in No Place to Hide, vol 3, no 1, April 2001, 'Special Issue on Russian and Ukrainian Research' by Arthur Firstenberg, editor of The Cellular Phone Taskforce.
61 Adapted from No Place To Hide, vol 3, no 1, April 2001, 'Special Issue on Russian and Ukrainian Research' by Arthur Firstenberg, editor of The Cellular Phone Taskforce.

Chapter 10

62 Professors Graeme Morgan, Royal North Shore, Robyn Ward, Prince of Wales and Michael Barton, Liverpool Hospital oncologists and radiotherapists of Sydney, conducted a study in 2004 regarding the debate on the funding and availability of cytotoxic drugs. The aim of the study was to answer questions about the contribution of curative or adjuvant cytotoxic chemotherapy to survival in adult cancer patients.
63 The advantage of local hyperthermia combined with conformal radiotherapy should be confirmed by a randomised phase 3 trial, comparing irradiation plus androgen suppression therapy with or without hyperthermia. *International Journal of Hyperthermia* 2007,

vol 23 no 5, pp 451–456 PMID: 17701536
64 Dr Jacobi van der Zee's paper titled 'Part 1: Clinical Hyperthermia' was reviewed in the *International Journal of Hyperthermia* March 2008 and presented at the Kadota Fund International Conference.
65 Further details can be found at radiowavebarlow.com.

Chapter 11
66 Some guidelines are even higher.
67 There would possibly be many more variables, such as the type of magnetic fields that are present and the assessment of the plumbing environment, etc.
68 The guide is for investigating two components of a dirty electrical environment only. To address all the frequencies and fields from 0Hz to 300 GHz is a vast area. For further information, The BioInitiative Report is available at www.bioinitiative.org
69 Huss et al 2007.

Chapter 12
70 Havas M, Rae W, Tel Oren A Ecopolitan 2009, www.ecopolitan.com/health-resources/emfprotection/147-health-effects-radio
71 *American Chronicle*, 23 April 2009. www.americanchronicle.com/articles/view/95811
72 Nikitina, V, p 9, 2003.
73 By order of the Head State Sanitary Physician of the Republic of Kazakhstan, 28 November 2003, r. No 69.
74 The author is currently compiling a list of the distributors in different countries. For purchase details, contact her at donnafisher@silentfields.com

Afterword
75 Compiled by participant in The BioInitiative Report Dr Henry Lai, PhD, Department of Bioengineering University

NOTES

of Washington, Seattle.

76 Cedric Garland, DPH (epidemiologist and adjunct prof). Department of Family and Preventive Medicine, Cancer Prevention and Control Program, University of California.

77 C K Wanebo and colleagues following on from Ian McKenzie 1965.

78 Wertheimer, N, Leeper. 'Adult cancer related to electrical wires near the home.' Int J Epidemiol 1982 11:345–355.

79 Erren in Stevens, Wilson, Anderson 1997, p 731.

Appendix D

80 For further information on the subject of lighting and health concerns refer to www.electricalpollution.com/documents/08_Havas_CFL_SCENIHR.pdf

81 Adapted from EMR and Health, 'How green is our lighting?' Jul–Sept 2007, Vol 3, No 3, page 9.

Appendix E

82 The signees of these resolutions have signed as individuals, giving their professional affiliations, but this does not necessarily mean this represents the views of their employers or their affiliated professional organisations. Excerpted from www.icems.eu